Essentials of Human Genetics

Second Editon

Edited by
Dr. Roopa Kulkarni
Senior Professor
Department of Anatomy
M.S. Ramaiah Medical College
Bangalore - 560054
and
Dr. R.N. Kulkarni
Professor & Head of the Department of Anatomy
M.S.U.G.E.F. International Medical School
M.S. Ramaiah Medical College Campus
Bangalore - 560054

PEEPEE
PUBLISHERS AND DISTRIBUTORS (P) LTD.

Essentials of Human Genetics

Published by
Pawaninder P. Vij and Anupam Vij

Peepee Publishers and Distributors (P) Ltd.
Head Office: 160, Shakti Vihar, Pitam Pura, Delhi-110 034 (India)
Correspondence Address:

7/31, First Floor, Ansari Road, Daryaganj
New Delhi-110 002 (India)
Ph: 65195868, 23246245, 9811156083
e-mail: peepee160@yahoo.co.in
e-mail: peepee160@rediffmail.com
e-mail: peepee160@gmail.com
www.peepeepub.com

First Edition: 2009

Second Edition Reprint: 2015

ISBN: 978-81-8445-118-4

Printed by :
BALAJI OFFSET PRINTERS, New Delhi-110035

Preface to Second Edition

The research in clinical genetics has been an excellent tool in solving many genetic disorders. To understand the newer concepts in the field, a basic knowledge in genetics is a must. Therefore a small effort has been made to simplify and compile the basic information in genetics.

The molecular level approach in diagnosing many diseases is becoming utmost essential for the correct treatment. Every day there are newer techniques in genetics to explore the most minute level. But for an undergraduate student, with a specified, limited duration of the study, it is not possible to keep up the advance information or update the information.

The basic principles behind the cell division and cell cycle have been included which are essential for understanding the genetic basis or cause for the diseases. It also gives an insight to the rationale behind genetic investigation.

Preface

It gives me immense pleasure in bringing this book, **'Essentials of Human Genetics'**.

The field of medical genetics has become the ultimate in the diagnosis of most of the diseases. Thus the human genetics has grown tremendously, beyond limits. But so much of information has overburdened the medical and paramedical students during their study period.

Thus the most challenging job in teaching Human Genetics to medical and paramedical students is to provide adequate information in a very short period of hours which are allocated to the field of genetics. At the same time make the subject easy and understandable by simple language and help the students to feel at ease even though this field of science is at length and complexity.

The Medical Council of India has reduced the duration of 1st MBBS course from one and half years to one year, giving less time for the students to study various branches in Anatomy apart from other subjects, therefore an effort is made to put most of the relevant information in Human Genetics in one concise book and facilitate students to refer to one book to save their time. The chapters which are arranged provide adequate, required information which helps the undergraduate and the postgraduate students to understand and remember the clinical genetics and create interest to acquire more knowledge in the field of medical genetics.

Most of the basic information like the normal cell division, Mendel's Law of Inheritance and variations have been excluded as these topics are studied at 10+2 level of education.

Acknowledgements

It gives us immense pleasure to thank the management of Gokula Education Foundation (Medical) for giving us an opportunity to serve in this prestigious institution and allow us to proceed with the academic activities.

Firstly, we would like to thank Mr. B.R. Prabhakara, CEO, Dr. K.N. Sharma, Executive Director, Gokula Education Foundation and Dr. Dua Sharma, Former Principal M.S. Ramaiah Medical College, Bangalore who have been a constant inspiration and encouragement for all the academic activities which helped us in bringing out this book.

We are highly obliged and thankful to Dr. S. Kumar, Principal and Dean, M.S. Ramaiah Medical College, Teaching and Memorial Hospitals, Bangalore, without whose support and constant encouragement, would have been a dream to bring out this book. His constant support and concern for students has motivated us to bring out this book **"Essentials of Genetics"**.

We also thank all our colleagues, staff and postgraduate students in the department who supported and motivated us.

We thank our family for giving us their time which we needed and stood by us throughout the process of preparation.

Last but not the least we sincerely thank Mr. Pawaninder P. Vij, Director of Peepee Publishers and Distributors to pen this maiden book from us.

Bangalore

Dr. Roopa Kulkarni
and
Dr. R.N. Kulkarni

Contents

1 Chapter INTRODUCTION

Genetics is that branch of medical science which deals with the study of hereditary material passing from one generation to another. It deals with heredity and variation. Genetics is studied in humans and plants (all living cells). The human genetics and plant genetics have been extensively studied. In agriculture, medicine and in society the genetics has developed greatly. During early 1900 there were greater, improved techniques in agriculture for selective breeding, higher yielding and destruction of insect pests and weed killers. Gradually, artificial insemination, embryo transfer, cloning, etc were introduced in animals to get desirable traits; e.g., required yield and butter fat of milk in cows and better quality and yield of wool in sheep. In case of human beings experiments were conducted in genetics to improve the angiogenesis which is useful in myocardial infarction, introduction of deficient amino acid in deficiencies of protein etc. For all these kind of growth the knowledge of genetics is very essential. Even though the genetics has a limited application as there is lack of corrective measures, and if there are any, they are very expensive, but still it is a boon for the sufferers and affordable.

Thus, the genetics deals with the study of 'GENES'.

- Genes are the basic units of heredity.
- Gene is a segment of DNA that determines the structure of an amino acid chain or polypeptide.
- Genes direct the process of protein synthesis. If one sequence is altered, the chain of events changes, leading to anomalies.
- Total genetic complement or make up is defined as "Genome".

- Genes are borne by the chromosomes in a linear series as parts of specific DNA molecule, each with its specific place and is called 'Gene locus'.

When we look back into the history, it was not known to the people how the reproduction took place and how the characteristics of the parents were transferred to the new offspring even though the reproduction and transmission of characteristic features of parents were taking place. It was thought that the male produced the offspring and it was the female who nursed in the womb and outside after birth.

There are such innumerable assumptions regarding the reproduction and transmission of parental characters to the offspring. It was only after the invention of the microscope the structure of the cells, the fertilization and reproduction came into light. The reproduction is the fusion of male and female cell components. Charles Darwin worked extensively on this fusion or blending of the male and female cells and stated that there is constant struggle for existence and survival of the fittest. Later on Gregor Mendel, who is one of the contemporary of Charles Darwin, came out with the answer. His theories explained how the characteristic features of the individuals resembled with parents or one of the parents, physically and also in behavior.

Gregor Mendel (1822–1884) was an Austrian monk who is also called 'Father of Modern Genetics'. The farmers and herders were breeding selectively the plants and animals to produce more useful plants and animals for thousands of years. But since the factors responsible for inheritance were not known to them it was not successful always. Gregor Mendel cultivated and tested the numerous pea plants and later conducted experiments in the reproduction of honey bees. In case of study on pea plants showed that one in four pea plants had pure breeds of recessive alleles, two of the four were hybrid and one of the four was dominant. He thus named these observations as laws of inheritance which consisted of:

1. Law of segregation; and
2. Law of independent assortment.

In law of segregation, a pair of alleles of each parent separate and only one allele passes from each parent to an offspring. The allele that is inherited from parents' pair of alleles is a matter of chance. This occurs during meiosis.

In law of independent assortment, different pairs of alleles are passed on to the offspring independently resulting in new combinations of genes present which were not present in either of the parents. For example, a particular eye colour does not increase or decrease the likelihood of having six digits in each hand. This is due to the fact that the genes for independently assorted traits are located on different chromosomes.

These two principles of inheritance, units of inheritance and dominance were the beginnings of modern genetics. But Mendel did not realize the exceptions to these laws or principles.

His work on honey bee reproduction was not successful as there was difficulty in controlling the mating behaviors of queen bee. By 1890 there were inventions of better microscopes and it was possible to study the cell division and sexual reproduction which helped in better study in genetics and Mendel's hypotheses in the field of genetics were retested. The hypotheses were rejected when Mendel was alive but they were accepted and further studies were conducted to confirm only after his death. There was evolution in the field of biology when the Mendelian genetics with Darwin's theory of natural selection were combined.

Mendel worked on garden pea plants because they could be grown easily in large numbers and also has male and female reproductive organs that help in self pollination along with pollination with other plants. He also could study many generations of these plants and conclude on the genetic inheritance. But his observations were after the experiments conducted in the laboratory; the hypotheses were not accepted initially.

His conclusions after the experiments conducted were:

1. The inheritance of each trait is determined by 'units' or 'factors' that are passed on to descendants unchanged. These units are now called 'GENES'.
2. An individual inherits one such unit from each parent for each trait.

3. A trait may not show up in an individual but can be passed on to the next generation.

GENETICS AND MEDICINE

The study of genetics started in 1900 by Gregor Mendel. In 20th century it took a big leap and gradually the disorders related to genes were identified. About more than 10,000 gene related disorders have been identified. Revolution in genetics and molecular biology has played an important role in medicine. Most of the disorders of cardiovascular system, endocrine system–especially the diabetes mellitus, psychiatry and cancers are linked to genetics.

Studies of hereditary patterns were seen in horses about 6000 years back in Babylonia. The study was documented and the patterns of transmission of body characters were recorded.

Hereditary transmission of body characters like baldness, obesity, height of the individual, polydactily, albinism were studied by Aristotle, Hippocrates and Pierre de Maupertius. Gradually, during the late 19th and 20th century there were lot of modifications, inventions and improvements in the techniques used in the medical research field that helped in recognizing many genetic disorders. Early identification and treatment for the disease has given greater life expectancy. The relation between genetics and environment and the interaction between both of them has manifested in heart disease and diabetes mellitus whenever there was non co-ordination between the two.

Spontaneous miscarriages (40–50% of the first trimester pregnancy termination), 2–3% of neonates have at least one major genetic disorder. In childhood, about 50% blind, 50% deaf children and 1% of malignancy have been linked to genetics. Watson and Crick's contribution to the molecular genetics is a great contribution to the field of molecular biology.

BRANCHES IN GENETICS

The genetic field has many sub-divisions or many branches. It started with study of genetics at cellular level and has almost extended at the molecular level. The branches are as follows:

1. **Cytogenetics:** This deals with the study of chromosomes which are obtained from dividing cells arrested at metaphase stage of cell

division. Earlier the cells from bone marrow were obtained for cytogenetic study as there were many dividing cells in the red bone marrow. Gradually there was use of phytohemagglutinin to separate red blood corpuscles from white blood corpuscles, which caused agglutination of red blood corpuscles. It was also observed that the white blood cells multiplied faster in presence of phytohemagglutinin–a pant origin. This was followed by the use of colchicine that arrested the cell division at metaphase.

2. **Biochemical genetics:** This was introduced to understand the concepts of inborn error of metabolism because the genetic anomalies occur due to the change in the enzyme (enzyme defect) or its effect (action of enzyme) on various metabolism in the body. It also helped in identifying dominant and recessive genes (affected individuals or sufferer and carriers) in both male and female individuals.
3. **Immunogenetics:** It started with the discovery of ABO blood groups, MN groups and Rh blood groups.
4. **Somatic cell genetics:** In this the cells are cultured and are stored for future use. There are cells called HeLa cells which are the cancer cells of cervical carcinoma. They are also named as immortal cell line. They are so named because they were obtained from a patient called Henrietta Lacks (HeLa) who died of her cancer in 1951. These cells were remarkably durable and proliferate extensively during the process of incubation and multiplication. These cells have been useful in studying cancer markers, testing polio vaccine, in studying the mode of infestation by parvo virus and many more research works. The somatic cell genetics thus has a big role in clarification of genetic basis of cancer.
5. **Molecular genetics:** This branch stated with the identification of DNA and use of artificially synthesized RNA consisting of only uracil. Addition of PCR was a major breakthrough in molecular genetics. This helped in cloning of cells. The cloned cells were used in gene therapy. This branch also helped in identifying the parents in disputed conditions and find out the criminals.
6. **Clinical genetics:** Clinical genetics is the medical speciality which deals with the practice of clinical medicine with particular attention

to hereditary disorders. The genetic disorders can be birth defects, delay in development, short stature, epilepsy, autism, dental defects, endocrine disorders etc. It involves two branches of genetics – one is diagnosis and the other is the genetic counseling. It is not only for the individuals but also for family members of the patient to explain the severity, risks involved and transmission to next generation.

The chromosomal disorders like deletion, inversion, translocations, trisomies of autosomes and sex chromosomes, monosomies of autosomes and sex chromosomes need to be attended specifically in genetics clinics. The scope of medical or clinical genetics includes many areas such as physicians for diagnosing/rule out genetic disorders, cytogenetic and biochemical laboratories and technicians, genetic counselors and nutritionists. Thus medical/clinical genetics is becoming more and more relevant and extensive field of study.

7. **Statistical genetics:** Due to extensive research in the field of genetics, after the Human Genome Project, there are lots of academic projects and commercial tasks in mapping all the human genome. The relation between disease and behavior is being found out using the measured genes or genetic markers. The study in population gives a varied response to disease causing agents and the genetic complement of that individual. This requires a sound statistical methodology for carrying our genetic linkage associated with the disorder. This study is called statistical genetics.
8. **Pharmacogenetics:** It is the study of differences in response to various drugs. The drug therapy in the routine disease management is based on pharmacogenetics. The responses to various drugs are different in different individuals and this is due to genetic variation affecting the metabolism, toxicity and efficacy. It deals with drug-gene interactions. It started as early as 1930. It is relevant to individual variation in drug response in two ways: 1. Variation in rate of absorption of the drug by the body, its metabolism, transportation and excretion of drug. It is called the variation in pharmacokinetics. 2. Variation affecting pharmacodynamics of the drug. It deals with the genetic causes of variability responding to drug which is due to genetic/allelic variation in targets like enzymes, receptors and metabolic pathways. There are three phenotypes

identified. They are: 1. Normal metabolizers; 2. Poor metabolizers; and 3. Fast or ultrafast metabolizers. Poor metabolizers are at risk because there is accumulation of the drugs to toxic levels due to slow metabolism of the drug. Fast or ultrafast metabolizers are probably being undertreated due to the fast metabolism leading to insufficient accumulation of therapeutic dose of the drug in tissues or blood. Therefore each individual responds to the same drug dosage in different ways. Therefore, like the individuals having a specific nucleotide chains in DNA and unique fingerprint pattern, there is unique response to the same drug and its dosage. Therefore, adverse drug reactions were reported along with the dosage information because it may be fatal in some cases (poor metabolizers) with the same therapeutic dose. The drug-gene interaction is also influenced by life style (modern life style changes), habits like cigarette smoking, drinking alcohol, diet, exposure to preservatives, food additives, taste enhancers, pesticides, fertilizers and environmental pollutants. The response to the therapeutic drug also depends on endogenous factors like age, gender, size of the body, state of health and disease and the rate of metabolism and excretion of the drug by the renal tubules and through the sweat glands. It is therefore one of the fast growing branches of genetics which deals with the study of enzyme activity, individual differences in drug response blood levels of drug, time and dose of the drug given, isolation of protein responsible for its action, synthesis of an antibody, isolation of mRNA and cDNA, identification of gene and finally to prove the genotype that responsible for the trait by correcting mutation in that gene.

9. **Pharmacogenomics:** It is defined as the study of interaction of drugs with the total genomes. Until 1998 the terminology was used in common with (was a part of) pharmacogenetics. Later this was separated from pharmacogenetics. All pharmacogenomic differences are polygenic and multifactorial which includes two or more major genes, dozens of modifier genes and environment. Some of the pharmacogeretic disorders are phenytoin-warfarin oxidation defects, G6PD deficiency, calcium channel defect etc.

There are various pharmacogenetics disorders and pharmacogenomic defects which exhibit ethnic differences, e.g., slow acetylator variant alleles are less in Japanese compared to Mediterranean people. Same in case of Asian and Caucasians for many of the drugs.

Thus, the study of pharmacogenetics and pharmacogenomics helps in increased therapeutic effects of drugs and reduced side effects. Thus helps in determining the accurate dosage of the therapeutic drug and prescription of drugs based on patient's genetic complement. It helps in synthesizing vaccines of genetic material and activation of immune system having benefits of existing vaccines with reduced side effects and risks of infections.

But these have limitations as there are many genes involved (20,000 genes) and each gene in each individual has to be studied for the treatment purpose which is a hilarious task. There is environmental effect which influences the genes and it again is difficult to change according to the climate, region and pollutants in that region. This may lead to expensive medicines which are specific to each individual. Ethnicity also is involved therefore it may be one of reasons for targeting a particular group or the race which may be very expensive but again it may not be applicable to the same racial population because they may not have the same genetic variation.

The pharmacogenomics has been applied extensively in the illnesses like cardiovascular disorders, attention deficit disorders, HIV, asthma, tuberculosis, diabetes, psychiatry and cancer.

10. **Population genetics:** It is the study of the frequency of occurrence of alleles within and between populations. It is closely related to evolutionary genetics because it depends heavily on challenges in gene frequencies.

Natural calamities can drastically reduce a population–usually unselective and results in genetic composition of small surviving population. Therefore is unlikely to be representative of original population.

Allele frequency: It is the relative abundance of an allele or genetic variant in a given population.

HOW DOES GENETIC STRUCTURE CHANGE?

Cause allele (genotype) frequencies through time by:

1. Mutation.
2. Migration.
3. Natural selection.
4. Genetic drift.
5. Nonrandom mating.

1. In mutation spontaneous change in DNA occurs which creates new alleles. It is the ultimate source of all genetic variation.
2. In migration, individuals move into population, introduce new alleles which leads to 'gene flow'.
3. In natural selection certain genotypes produce more offspring, differences in survival or reproduction leads to differences in fitness; that leads to adaptation, e.g., resistance to antibacterial soap is different in different generations. Natural selection can cause populations to diverge other selection or sickle cell allele.
4. **Genetic drift:** Genetic change can by chance alone–sampling errors occur due to misrepresentation and small populations.
5. **Nonrandom mating:** Mating combines alleles into genotypes. Nonrandom mating leads to nonrandom allele combinations.

The reproduction of any organism including mankind is not only interlocked with its environment but also gives rise to a new life. Therefore the study of formation of a new individual is called–reproduction.

There are two types of reproductions: 1. Asexual or vegetative 2. Sexual reproduction where there is WELDING of half of the genetic memory of two parents and formation of a new individual of its kind.

For sexual reproduction there are certain specialized reproductive cells with rearrangement of genetic material and reduction to a half the quantity found in general cells of the body. The two reproductive cells–one from each parent, approach and fuse, restore the somatic genetic material and grow to give rise to new individual of its kind.

Sexual reproduction is divided into several stages–Gametogenesis, Fertilization, Cleavage, Gastrulation and Organogenesis.

During the reproductive phase the growth, morphogenetic movement, patterned differentiation, regional degeneration and apoptosis (programmed cell death) take place.

During prenatal development, cells undergo repeated division, mature and differentiate in structure and function. Finally they either lose ability to divide (as in neurons) or persist as stem cells capable of dividing throughout life (as in case of hemopoietic tissue of bone marrow).

Facts: Rate of cell division varies in different tissues:

- It depends on mechanical stress, demand for secretion, absorption or injury. (Coupled with demand for growth and replacement). If there is faulty coupling–either cell fail to grow or overgrow (neoplasms).
- Compounds called CHALONES inhibit cell division. But when cells are destroyed chalones are inhibited, cells grow fully and chalones levels are restored which again inhibit the cell growth.

The interphase lasts for 12 to 24 hours in mammalian cells.

During interphase the cell is:

- Constantly synthesizing RNA.
- Produce protein.
- Grow in size.

Two types of cell divisions: 1. Mitosis 2. Meiosis.

The living organisms are dynamic, homeostasis is preserved despite short term fluctuations in the surroundings.

[Homeostasis–regulation and maintenance of body temperature, blood pressure, hydration, osmolarity, electrolyte and hydrogen ion concentration, glucose and oxygen levels, endocrine secretory control systems, varying rates of cell growth death and replacement, behavioral patterns rearing of the young, searching and procuring food and shelter etc.]

Cell growth starts from the life inside the womb or uterus. The intrauterine and extrauterine growth is called EMBRYOLOGY.

The reproduction of any organism including mankind is not only interlocked with its environment but also gives rise to a new life. Therefore the study of formation of a new individual is called– reproduction.

There are two types of reproductions:

1. Asexual or vegetative.
2. Sexual reproduction where there is WELDING of half of the genetic memory of two parents and formation of a new individual of its kind.

For sexual reproduction there are certain specialized reproductive cells with rearrangement of genetic material and reduction to a half the quantity found in general cells of the body. The two reproductive cells–one from each parent, approach and fuse, restore the somatic genetic material and grow to give rise to new individual of its kind.

Sexual Reproduction

During the reproductive phase of the growth, morphogenetic movement, patterned differentiation, regional degeneration and apoptosis (programmed cell death) take place.

Cell Division: It is the reproduction of the CELLS.

During prenatal development, cells undergo repeated division, mature and differentiate in structure and function. Finally they either lose ability to divide (as in neurons) or persist as stem cells capable of dividing throughout life (as in case of hemopoietic tissue of bone marrow).

Before the cells divide each cell passes through a cycle consisting of various stages of growth, resting and replication.

Cell Cycle: The sequence of activities exhibited by the cells is called cell cycle.

It consists of two broad phases:

1. Interphase.
2. Mitotic phase (M-phase).

The interphase lasts for 12 to 24 hours in mammalian cells. During interphase the cell is:

- Constantly synthesizing RNA.
- Produce protein.
- Grow in size.

Depending upon molecular events in cells the interphase is divided into FOUR steps. They are G0 (Gap Zero), G1 (Gap One), S (Synthesis) and G2 (Gap Two).

G0: Cell does not enter into cycle. Stops dividing. It is a temporary resting phase. It may be a permanent as in case of neurons.

G1: • Cells increase in size.

- Produce more RNA.
- Synthesize protein.

There is a protein called P53 which is tumor suppressor protein. It binds to specific DNA sequence called 'GUARDIAN OF GENOME' and it controls the cell cycle to enable repair of damaged DNA activation of cell cycle control mechanism at this stage. If everything is functioning normally and any damage to the DNA has been corrected the cell moves on through the cell cycle. If something is wrong, the cycle halts and apoptosis (cell death) takes place.

P53 is mutated in skin and colorectal cancers. Here the cell cycle clock spins out of control.

S: Synthesis of DNA takes place (Replication of DNA).

At the end of S phase of cell cycle there is a check point where the cyclic AMP inhibits synthesis of DNA. The period between end of S phase and beginning of G2 phase it is the check point.

G2: In this phase cell produces more protein. The cell double checks the duplicated chromosomes for error, making any needed repair. G2 phase has a check point and it ensures the cell is ready to complete cell division.

M: It lasts for about 1 to 2 hours. Cell growth and protein production stop. All the energy of the cell is focused on complex and orderly division into two similar daughter cells. The M-phase is further divided into many sub-phases called–PROPHASE, METAPHASE, ANAPHASE and TELOPHASE.

Cell Clock in the cell cycle. It is the executive decision maker. It integrates the regulatory signals received by the cell with current state of health of the cell.

Two events occur in cell division:

1. Division of the nucleus (Karyokinesis); and
2. Division of the cytoplasm (Cytokinesis).

Nuclear division takes place by three ways:

1. Amitosis 2. Mitosis 3. Meiosis.

Amitosis

Amitosis is the DIRECT division of the cell where there is random distribution of nuclear material to the resulting daughter cells. But this kind of division takes place rarely in cartilage cells. This type of cell division also takes place in pathological conditions.

The mitosis and meiosis are INDIRECT cell divisions.

Among the two types the meiosis consists of two stages. Stage I and Stage II.

Mitosis

1. Occurs in somatic cells.
2. Results in the distribution of identical copies of parent cells' genomes.
3. DNA synthesized during 'S' phase of interphase and is doubled leading to half the number of chromosomes to the daughter cells.
4. It consists of four sub phases–PROPHASE, METAPHASE, ANAPHASE and TELOPHASE.

Prophase

a. Strands of chromatin begin to shorten and thicken.
b. Chromatin strands resolve into recognizable chromosomes – Two chromatids and centromere.
c. Centrioles separate outside the nucleus and move in opposite direction.

d. Parallel microtubules are synthesized between centrioles and create central spindles. Other tubules radiate from centriole to form astral rays or asters [Spindle along with two asters form achromatic figure called DIASTER or AMPHIASTER].

e. Nucleoli disappear.

f. Nuclear envelop disintegrates into small vesicles.

Metaphase

a. Nuclear envelop disappears.

b. Spindle microtubules invade central region of cell.

c. The imaginary plane where chromosomes are arranged is called metaphase plate or equatorial plate.

d. Chromosomes attach to spindle microtubules at centromeres and appear as star like ring when viewed from the poles.

Anaphase

a. Double structured centromere halves to separate the chromatids. Lengthwise split into 2 new chromosomes.

b. The chromosomes move apart – one to each pole, by the action of microtubules influenced by addition of tubulin.

c. Cleavage furrow appears in the cell cytoplasm and membrane.

Telophase

a. Diploid numbers of chromosomes are given to each cell.

b. Nuclear membrane reappears.

c. Nucleoli reappear.

d. Cytoplasmic division begins with distribution of mitochondria and other organelles.

e. Cleavage furrow deepens to divide the cell into two – the cytoplasm which condenses due to deepening of the furrow is called MID BODY where the dense microtubules and microfilaments if actin and myosin are seen. Eventually the cells separate due to the deepening of the furrow which is due to appearance of actin and myosin microfilaments and their contraction at the site of the furrow helps in deepening of the furrow and separation of cells.

f. Spindle remnant disappears.

Mechanism of cell division is controlled by:

A. Local factors B. Endocrine secretion.

A. The Local factors: Diffusion of metabolites from one cell group to another which stimulates or inhibits the activity.

B. Endocrine secretions like Somatotrophic hormone, Progesterone, Thyroxin, Corticosteroids, Cyclic AMP (Adenosine Mono Phosphate).

Applied Anatomy

Disruption of mitosis is by:

1. **Colchicine and Its Derivatives:** Inhibit or reverse spindle microtubule formation and arrest cell division at metaphase. This is made use in cytogenetic to study chromosomes.
2. **Ionizing Radiation:** It causes non-disjunction or lagging of chromatids leading to aneuploidy. Radiation may damage the cell and inhibit mitosis altogether. Failure of the epithelia to replace the lost cells with consequent ulceration of the skin and the mucous membrane occurs when the epithelia are exposed to ionizing radiation. It is called RADIATION SICKNESS.

Meiosis

This type of cell division takes place in gonadal (gametogenic) cells.

In the interphase, prior to the cell division, there is replication of DNA (tetraploid DNA).The number of chromosomes is double (diploid).

There are two stages – MEIOSIS I and MEIOSIS II.

Meiosis I

DNA is reduced to half the amount. Chromosome number is reduced to half (haploid).

It consists of five sub-phases. They are–LEPTOTENE, ZYGOTENE, PACHYTENE, DIPLOTENE and DIAKINESIS.

Leptotene: Chromosomes appear as individual threads attached at one end to the nuclear envelop and show characteristic beads

(Chromomeres) throughout their length. DNA replication has occurred in preceding S-phase.

Zygotene: Chromosomes come together side by side in homologous pairs. Homologous chromosomes pair point for point progressively beginning at the attachment to nuclear envelop. This process is called SYNAPSIS, CONJUGATION OR PAIRING. Ultra-microscopically appear as SYNAPTONEMAL COMPLEX. Each pair of bivalent chromosomes further shortens.

Pachytene: Shortening, thickening, followed by spirally of the chromosomes. The chromatids joined at centromere become visible. Bivalent pair is tetrad with four chromatids – two chromatids from each bivalent chromosome, partially coil round each other. During this stage there is exchange of DNA occurs by breaking and rejoining of strands facilitated by the synaptonemal complex.

Diplotene: Further shortened, homologous pairs, separate except where there is crossing. Chromatids and chiasmata appear.

Diakinesis: Centromeres separate further with adhesion of exchanged segments. Nucleoli disappear. Asters and spindles appear. Nuclear envelop disappears. Chromosomes move towards equatorial plate.

2 Chapter CHROMOSOMES

Derived from Greek: **Chroma** is color and **soma** is body.

Chromosomes are the deeply stained thread like bodies or structures within the nucleus of each animal cell.

They are **composed of DNA, Histones (basic proteins), Nonhistones (acidic proteins) and small amount of RNA.** This material of chromosome in the nucleus is called the 'Chromatin network'.

Individual chromosomes are visualized microscopically, only during the cell division at **metaphase**.

Each chromosome presents a primary constriction called **centromere** and two pairs of arms– one pair is proximal or short and is called the 'p' arm (p stands for petit which means small or short). The other arm is the distal or the long arm and is called 'q' arm ('q' i.e., 'g' that stands for grand or great or big arm). These arms are called the **chromatids.** The tips of the chromatids are called the **telomeres**.

The position of the centromere varies in different chromosomes.

1. When the centromere is in the middle, with p and q arms equal in length, such chromosome is called METACENTRIC.
2. When centromere is located at some distance from the mid point- with short p arms and long q arms it is called SUBMETACENTRIC.
3. If the centromere is near the end of 'p' arm it is called acrocentric (NOT telocentric).
4. When the centromere is at the end, it is called telocentric (NOT acrocentric).

In acrocentric chromosome p arm is absent.

In humans, telocentric chromosomes are absent.

In some chromosomes there will be a secondary constriction in the p arm and the part of the p arm distal to the secondary constriction is called **satellite body**. The chromosomes having the satellite bodies are called SAT CHROMOSOMES.

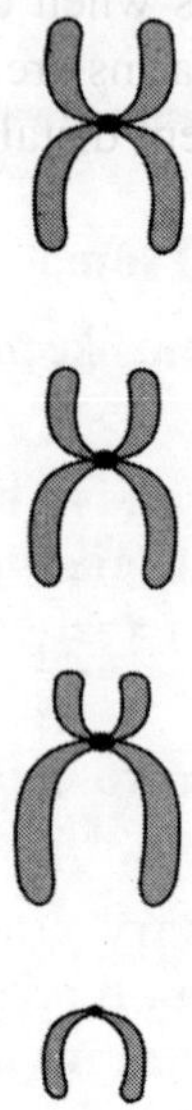

Fig. 2.1: Types of chromosomes

The total number of chromosomes is constant in that species.

Human somatic cells and immature or premature germ cells contain 46 chromosomes. This number is called the **'diploid number'**. They contain 44 or 22 pairs of AUTOSOMES and 2 or 1 pair of SEX CHROMOSOMES. The autosomes are responsible for the body characters and the sex chromosomes are for the sexual characters of an individual.

In mature germ cells the number is 23 chromosomes (half the diploid) therefore it is called the **'haploid number'**.

The sex chromosomes in female are homologous pair and they are

XX. In male the sex chromosomes are heterologous and are XY. They are unequal.

In female, out of the two X chromosomes, one is highly coiled and the other is highly uncoiled. The highly coiled is genetically inactive and becomes active only during cell division and fertilization. It exhibits in the somatic cell as BARR BODY.

The "Y" chromosome is in male cells, detected as an intensely fluorescent body within the nucleus of cells when cells are stained with fluorochrome dyes. The tips of the 'q' arms are very bright and are identified by this feature. Such fluorescent distal ends are called 'F' bodies.

3 Chapter BARR BODY

It is a highly coiled, heterochromatic, inactive X chromosome, appears as a plano convex body in the nucleus of the cell attached to the nuclear envelope.

The cells which exhibit Barr body are– the superficial epithelial cells of buccal mucosa. These were first noted by Barr and Bertram in 1949.This is synthetically an inert body. These are also seen in mature white blood cells (polymorphonuclear leucocytes) of females. The inert X chromosome appears as 'drum stick' like projection from the edges of the nuclear lobes which are irregular. They are very well demarcated in 3% of cells (Range is 1 to 17%). Lyon stated that the inert X chromosome does not get involved in synthetic activity. During cell division it undergoes methylation and becomes active. It is the euchromatic, lightly stained, active X chromosome which is involved in protein synthesis. This is called Lyonization/Lyon hypothesis (Lyon 1962).

The inert X chromosome also replicates later during interphase.

The number of Barr bodies is equal to the total number of X chromosomes minus 1.

(n= X-1 where n= number of Barr body, X is the number of X chromosomes).

Therefore in normal male n= 1, therefore 1x-1= 0 (there is no Barr body in normal male).

In normal female n=2X-1=1 i.e. there is one Barr body.

If Barr body is seen in the epithelial cell nucleus of buccal smear of male there will be 2X chromosomes along with Y chromosome (47 XXY- Klinefelter's syndrome).

XXXY will have two Barr bodies; XXX will have again two Barr bodies in their epithelial cells.

Thus the total number of Barr bodies helps us to know the total number of X chromosomes in the given epithelial cell.

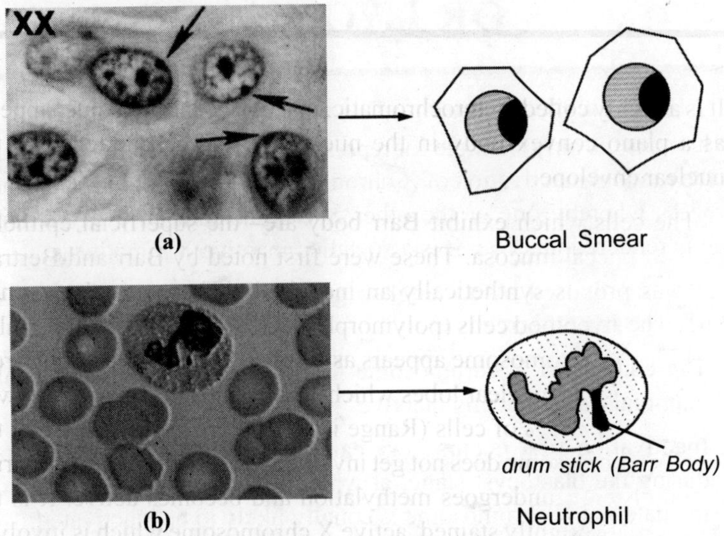

Fig. 3.1: Arrows indicate the Barr body in epithelial cell and neutrophil.

4 Chapter LYON HYPOTHESIS OR LYON THEORY OR LYONISATION

In humans the only example for repression and depression mechanism is the random inactivation of X chromosome. Lyonisation is a normal process whereby one or the other X chromosome in every female cell is rendered inactive. It is also called inactive X hypothesis.

It was proposed by an English geneticist, Dr. Mary F. Lyon in 1961. The hypothesis says:

1. The condensed X chromosome found in cells of normal female mammals is genetically inactive.
2. Inactivation first occurs very early in embryonic development, during the blastocyst stage, at which time either the maternal or the paternal X chromosome is equally likely to be inactivated.
3. This inactivation event occurs independently and randomly in each blastocyst cell, but once the decision is made for a given cell, same X chromosome will be inactivated in all its descendent cells, thereby producing a clone from each of the original cell. The effect of this whole process is called 'Lyonisation'. It is to equalize the phenotypes in males and females. This phenomenon is known as dosage compensation. Although normal females possess twice as many X chromosomes as males, they generally have the same number of active X linked genes and the same amount of X linked gene products.

Experiments were conducted for the evidence in cats– calico and tortoise shell– whose patches in the fur are black or orange. Because humans lack fur, this cannot be compared to cats and also most of the calico cats are females. Therefore the best trait is phenotypic expression of the recessive X linked trait– anhydrotic ectodermal dysplasia. The affected males lack sweat glands, teeth and most of their body hair. Described by Charles Darwin as the 'toothless men of Schinde'. Studies of females heterozygous for this gene reveal considerable variability in phenotypic expression taking the form of irregular skin patches with few or no sweat glands and some regions of the jaw with missing teeth or defective teeth. Many other human X linked genes are also known to show mosaic expression in heterozygous females.

X linked gene is for controlling the production of an enzyme-glucose 6- phosphate dehydrogenase (G6PD). But the human female who has 46,XX chromosomes has no more G6PD production compared to 46,XY, 46,XXY (Klinefelter) and 47XXX females. This suggests that regardless of how many X chromosomes are present in a given cell; only one X chromosome is active.

Therefore, the conclusion is that any X linked gene in an XX mammalian cell, only one of the two alleles remains active. There is a selective turning 'on' and 'off' of autosomal genes and also parental imprinting. Inactive X replicates later in the cell cycle than do the other chromosomes. X inactivation starts and spreads out from an X inactivation centre in the long arm near centromere-a gene called XIST– has been found. The exact method/steps during X inactivation and what prevents X inactivation of all X chromosomes is unknown. One of the causes for X inactivation is methylation of cytosine bases in DNA. X inactivation probably occurs as early as 16th day of IUL when the embryo consists of less than 5000 cells. Inactivation of X chromosome occurs only in somatic cell but not in germ cell. Therefore if X chromosome which is left over contains mutant gene-manifest carrier.

Whole chromosome except short arm containing Xg and steroid sulphatase (SO_4ase) (icthyosis) loci is not activated.

Some of the theories/additional twists in X chromosome inactivation:

1. Part of the X chromosome is not inactivated. These genes would be expressed doubly in normal females and in Klinefelter males (both with two X chromosomes). This, may be, there are additional X linked genes that escape inactivation.

2. Germ cells behave differently–In female fetuses future germ cells undergo Lyonisation along with somatic cells. But as the germ cells develop into oocytes and enter meiosis, their inactivated X chromosomes become reactivated. Thus each egg cell ends up with an active X. In males, the X chromosome undergoes precocious condensation in all primary spermatocytes just as they enter meiosis. But this is poorly understood and may not be true Lyonisation.
3. Some genes get reactivated as mammals age. But this was proved only in calico cats and mice.

X chromosome inactivation is perhaps the first and best known example of unexpected phenomenon that explains ambiguous pattern of gene expression.

Mapping primate genes– X chromosome is remarkably constant in size, banding patterns and gene content, not only among primates, but also among all the mammals that have been studied. E.g., the G6PD gene is X linked in most of the mammals including rat, mouse, cat, dog, cow, sheep, pig, mink, rabbit, kangaroo, donkey, horse as well as in seven primates which have been surveyed. Reason is not known.

5 Chapter KARYOTYPING

It is the characteristic chromosomal constitution. It is a study done to map out the chromosomes of an individual and arrange them in order.

METHOD OF PREPARATION OF CHROMOSOMES

It is called the cytogenetic study.

TISSUES PREFERRED

Skin, bone marrow cells, WBCs of peripheral blood, fibroblasts, amniotic fluid cells, chorionic villus cells etc.

The most preferred tissue is the WBCs of the peripheral blood.

Procedure: About 1 to 2 ml of blood is drawn in a heparinised syringe. Heparin is an anticoagulant. This blood is cultured in the medium prepared by the calf serum. Then it is treated with Phytohemaglutinin (PHA) which is extracted from red kidney beans.

PHA stimulates the WBCs to proliferate by mitosis. The cells are kept for 3 days at 37 degrees C. The WBCs are then collected by centrifugation and sedimentation method and transferred to culture bottles. The culture medium is mixed with streptomycin and penicillin to prevent growth and multiplication of bacteria.

Then colchicine is added to the culture bottles containing multiplying WBCs and kept for 2 hours. Colchicine arrests cell division at metaphase. The cells are collected by centrifugation, treated with hypotonic solution, fixatives are added and incubated for 20 minutes. Treating with hypotonic solution allows the cells to swell and to disperse the chromosomes. The most common fixative used is ethanol and acetic acid. The cells are gently shaken or small cell suspension is dropped on the sterile slide. The cells on the slide are allowed to dry at room temperature and stained with GEIMSA stain for conventional study. Proper chromosomal spread is selected, photographed and prints of enlarged pictures of chromosomal spread are obtained. Then photographs of the individual chromosomes are cut and arranged according to their size and position of centromere into homologous pairs – they are arranged in sequence– metacentric first, followed by submetacentric, telocentric and acrocentric.

Thus they are classified into 7 groups– 'A' to 'G'. This classification is called Denver's classification as it was decided in a place called Denver where all geneticists met during the conference in 1960 and accepted the classification. It is as follows:

A. 1to 3 pairs of autosomes– long and metacentric.

B. 4 & 5 pairs of autosomes– long and submetacentric.

C. 6 to 12 pairs of autosomes and X chromosome–medium and submetacentric.

D. 13 to 15 pairs of autosomes – long and acrocentric.

E. 16 to 18 pairs autosomes – short and submetacentric.

F. 19 & 20 pairs of autosomes – short and metacentric.

G. 21 & 22 pairs of autosomes and Y-chromosome – small and acrocentric.

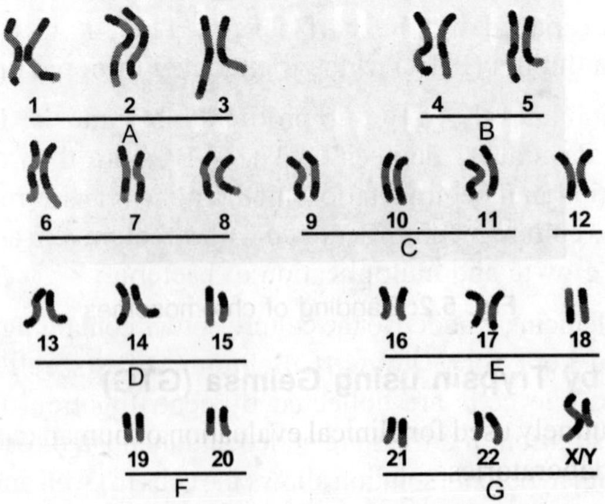

Fig. 5.1: Classification of chromosomes

BANDING TECHNIQUES

1. Q – BANDING (QUINACRINE MUSTARD).
2. G – BANDING (GIEMSA & TRYPSIN TREATMENT).
3. R – BANDING (REVERSAL G – BANDING – GIEMSA STAIN AFTER PREHEATING OF CHROMOSOMES TO 87°C).
4. C – BANDING (PRETREATMENT WITH ACID FOLLOWED BY ALKALI PRIOR TO GIEMSA STAIN).

Q-bands by fluorescence using Quinacrine (QFQ).

- It was the first banding technique to be discovered (Capersson in 1970).
- Used for studying the heteromorphism associated with chromosome 3, 4, acrocentric chromosomes and y chromosomes.
- Some of these are used as chromosome markers to identify the parental origin of additional chromosomes in trisomies and in paternity studies.

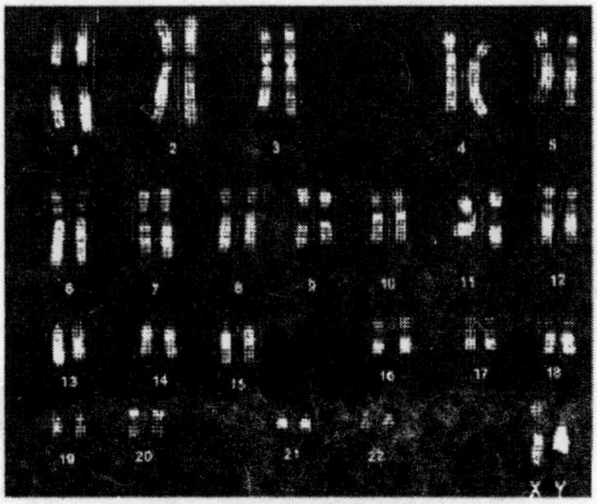

Fig. 5.2: Banding of chromosomes

G-bands by Trypsin using Geimsa (GTG)

- Most routinely used for clinical evaluation of human chromosomes in most laboratories.
- G-bands obtained are superior in resolution to those using flurochromes.

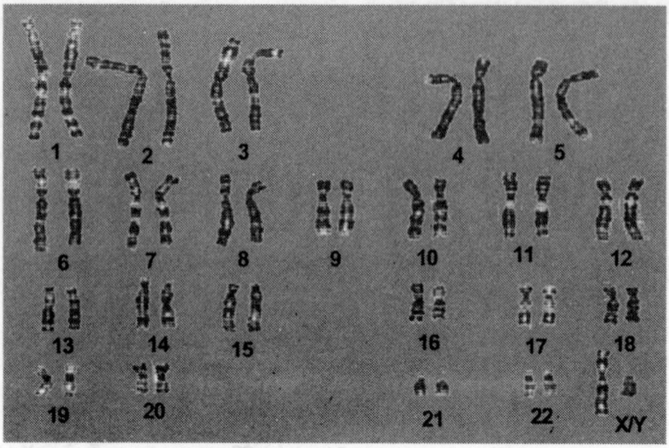

Fig. 5.3: G-banding of chromosomes

R-bands by Heat using Geimsa (RHG)

R-banding stains telomeric regions of chromosome more distinctively and is often useful for the study of structural changes involving chromosome ends that might go undetected with Q or G-banding.

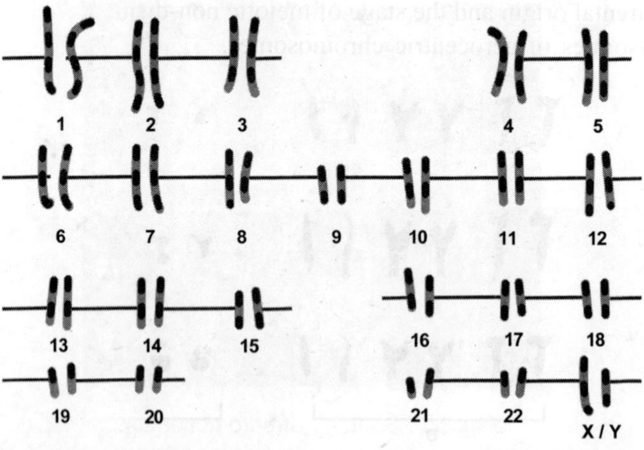

Fig. 5.4: R-banding of chromosomes

C-banding

Translocations involving the c-band region could be thoroughly investigated with c-banding to identify the precise translocation break points and to evaluate the status of centeromeric region.

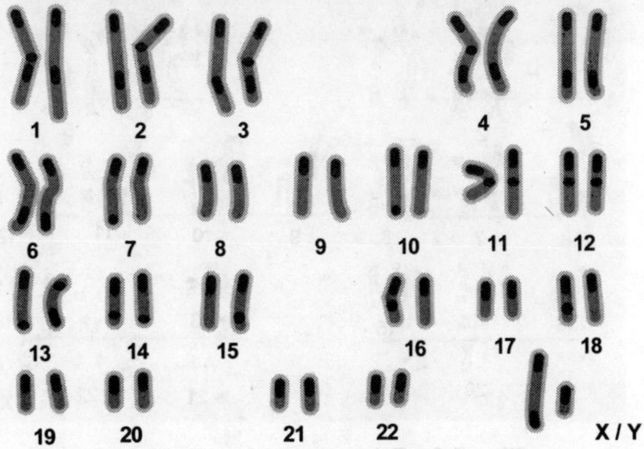

Fig. 5.5: C-banding of chromosomes

Nucleous Organizing Region (NOR)-bands

- They are stained by silver impregnation technique called as Ag-NOR banding.
- NOR- bands together with Q-bands have been used to identify parental origin and the stage of meiotic non-disjunction in human trisomies of acrocentric chromosomes.

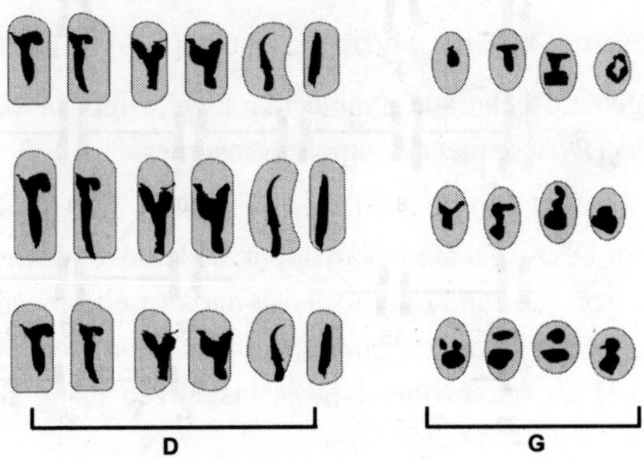

Fig. 5.6: Banding in chromosomes

High Resolution Banding

- Performed using prometaphase and prophase chromosomes.
- They facilitate better chromosomal analysis and used for resolving chromosomal abnormalities in leukemias.

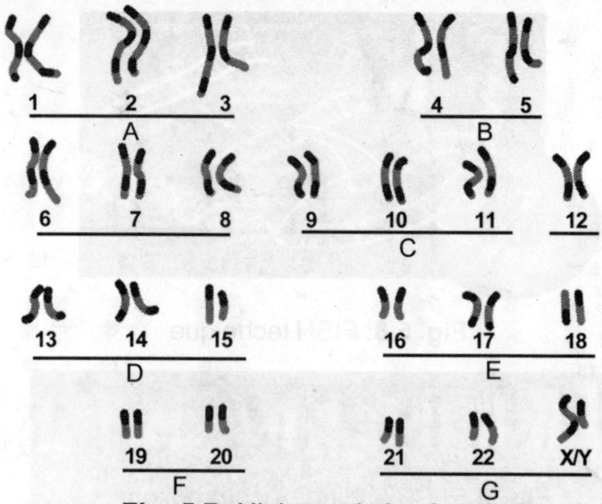

Fig. 5.7: High resolution banding

Anti-Kinetocore Antibody Banding

- Patients with scleroderma of CREST variety have auto antibodies to the kinetocore.
- Enables us to make out the kinetocore and centromere and follow its course thought the mitotic cycle.

Fluorescence In-Situ Hybridization (FISH) Technique

It is a cytogenetic technique at molecular level, which helps in locating the specific DNA sequences on chromosomes.

In this method, fluorescent probes, which are nothing but the fragments of DNA that are isolated, purified and amplified, are used. These DNA probes bind only to those parts of chromosomes which have high degree of sequence similarity. This fluorescent probe, bound to specific DNA on chromosome is visualized using fluorescence microscope.

In this method the probe has to be constructed and it must be large enough to hybridize with its target. The tagging is done using PCR (Polymerase Chain Reaction) with nucleotides and nick translation.

Therefore this method helps in identifying the structural abnormalities of chromosomes and the lost DNA on the chromosomes.

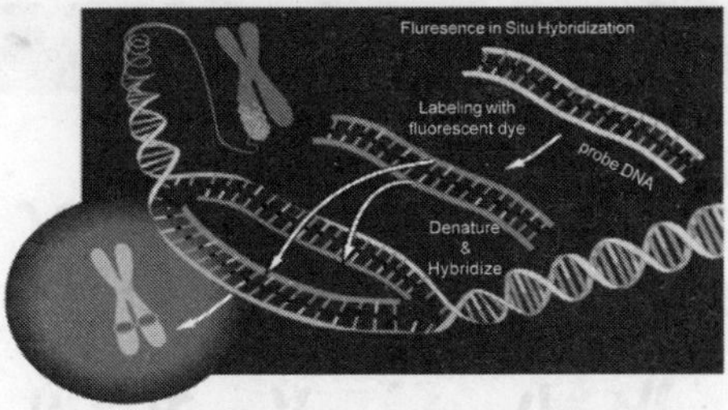

Fig. 5.8: FISH technique

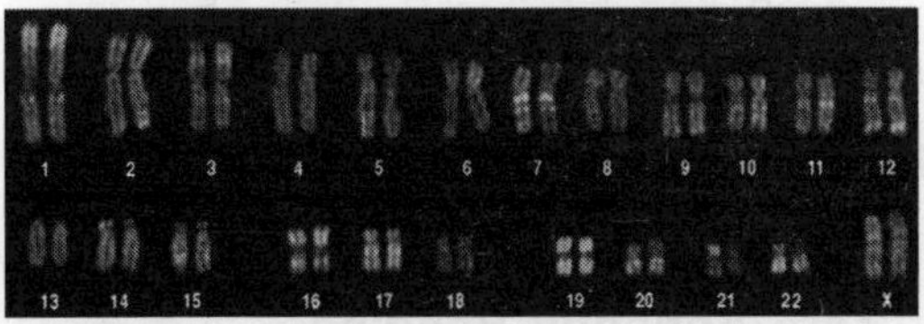

Fig. 5.9: Banding by FISH technique

Spectral Karyotyping (SKY)

It is a cytogenetic technique at molecular level, done to visualize all the chromosomes which appear painted in different colours. The DNA probes, which are fluorescently labelled specifically for each chromosome, are used. These labelled or coloured chromosomes are visualized using the fluorescence microscope. The number of DNA probes giving different colours are limited, therefore, a combination of various methods are used to visualize by using software which helps to paint each chromosome in different colours.

This technique is useful in identification of structural abnormalities.

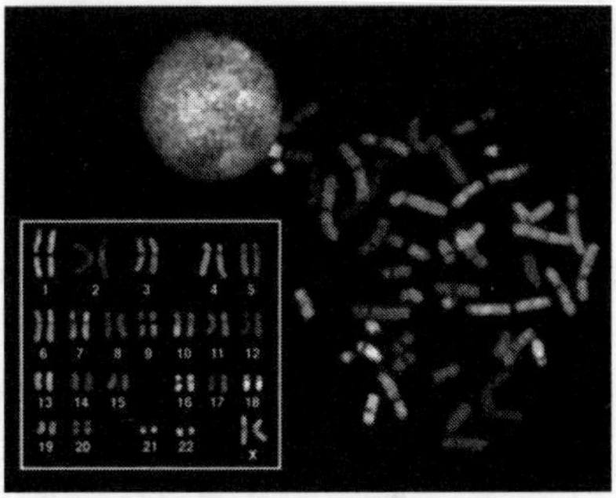

Fig. 5.10: Chromosomes with SKY technique

6 Chapter DNA (DEOXYRIBONUCLEIC ACID)

These are the fine filaments present in the chromosomes. In human 6.5 X 106 DNA is present in each somatic cell nucleus.

DNA consists of two parallel molecular chains running in positive directions in the form of double helix which is 25 nm in diameter. This double helix is a thin thread like flexible ladder.

The DNA and RNA are the macromolecules (polymers) composed of 3 units.

They are:

1. Fine carbon sugar.
2. Nitrogen containing base.
3. Phosphate.

The fine carbon sugar consists of:

a. Deoxyribose in DNA

b. Ribose in RNA

Nitrogen containing bases are:

a. Purines

b. Pyrimidines

Purines are:

i. Adenine (A)

ii. Guanine (G)

Pyrimidines are:

i. Thymine (T)

ii. Cytosine (C).

In RNA Uracil (U) Replaces Thymine

Phosphates are in the form of phosphoric acid.

The structural model of DNA consisting of right handed double helix was proposed by James Watson and Francis Crick, in 1953 and is termed as 'Watson and Crick' double helix model.

DNA is like a twisted ladder with vertical supports and horizontal rungs. The vertical supports are deoxyribose sugar and phosphate backbone (S=sugar and P=phosphate) vertically and alternately arranged. The horizontal rungs are arranged which are projecting inwards from each sugar and are formed by the pair of bases. Thus purine is connected to pyrimidine by hydrogen bonds, i.e., Adenine is connected to Thymine (A to T or T to A) and Cytosine connected to Guanine (C to G or G to C).

It is the lengthwise base sequences that provide all the genetic information within the DNA molecule. One purine or pyrimidine base linked to sugar is one nucleotide.

Nucleotides function as chemical 'Letters' which join to form 'Words'. Therefore a 'Gene' is a sequence of nucleotides making a word providing a chemical set of instructions making a specific protein

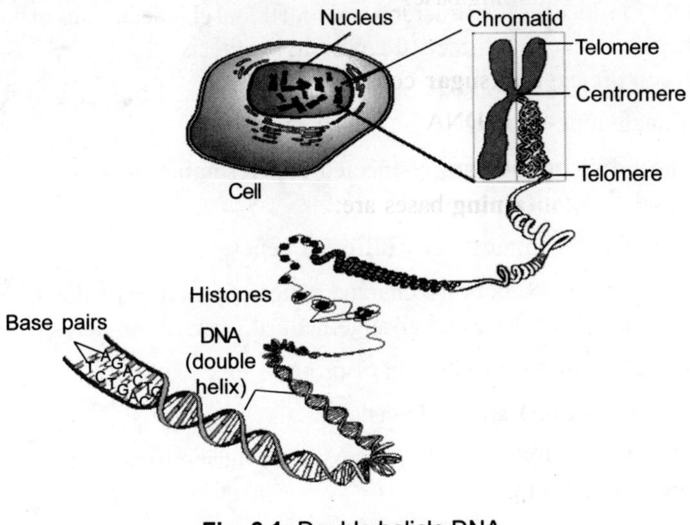

Fig. 6.1: Double helicle DNA

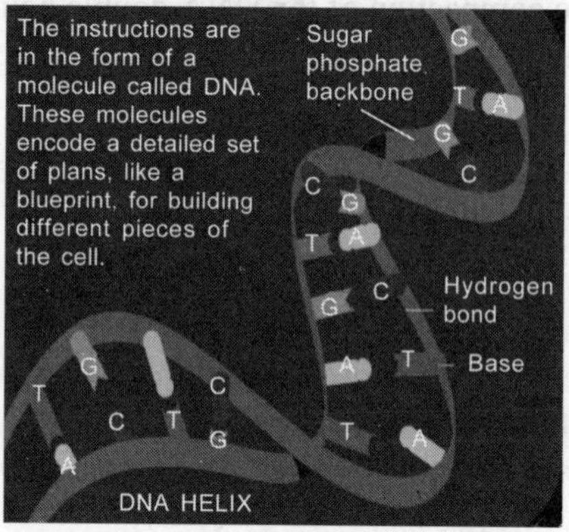

Fig. 6.2: Structure of DNA

A sequence is a coded message; therefore a gene is a segment of DNA molecule with a unique sequence of thousands of bases that tells the cell how to make a particular protein.

Each chromosome contains just one very long molecule of DNA stretched out. The total DNA in a single gamete (ovum or sperm) measures about ONE METER (3.28 ft.)

DNA contains information that directs the protein synthesis.

DNA influences the structural and functional characteristics of entire organism because it directs the protein synthesis.

DNA molecule consists of nucleotides – joined together to form two nucleotide strands.

These two strands are connected and resemble a twisted ladder (twisted along its long axis).

Each DNA contains many different genes.

Structural and functional characteristics of proteins are determined by the kinds, numbers and arrangement of their amino acids.

DNA directs the production of proteins in 2 steps:

1. Transcription and 2. Translation.

The DNA double helix starts separating during transcription by an enzyme called helicase.

There are histone and non-histone proteins in the chromosomes which help in the compaction of the DNA double helix cell division. During cell division, the DNA fiber continues to condense and at metaphase about 10,000 fold compaction takes place.

In cells the information encoded in DNA helps to direct the development and maintenance of the organism.

Chapter 7

MITOCHONDRIAL DNA (mt DNA)

Mitochondrion is an organelle which is a powerhouse of a cell.

Mitochondrion has a small amount of DNA – consisting of circular molecules of 16569 nucleotides each.

The mitochondrial DNA is relatively easy to purify and its simple structure makes it ideal for some types of analysis.

Although each individual has over a trillion cells, each cell has several hundred mitochondria, each mitochondrion has about 10 copies of DNA circle, virtually all of the over $\mathbf{10^{15}}$ molecules of mtDNA within a person seem to be identical.

Ovum has mitochondria in its cytoplasm and sperm head is only nuclear part of the cell, therefore when zygote is formed, the cytoplasm of the ovum takes part and its mitochondria are also included in the zygote. Thus genes in mtDNA follow an exclusively maternal inheritance pattern, generation after generation.

The mutation rate of mtDNA is much higher than that of nuclear DNA. Mitochondrial DNA is thus a sensitive indicator of evolutionary modification that can lead to racial differences.

The mitochondrial DNA ancestor has to be a woman, of course, since mitochondria are transmitted only by females.

Mitochondrial DNA is now being used for many studies of migrations and origins. But disagreements are spirited among and between archeologists, anthropologists, linguists, molecular biologists and others.

The absence of pure races is also due to the population intermixtures that result from migration.

Gene flow is not just a recent phenomenon. Fossils increasingly indicate that several different forms of homosepiens coexisted ten thousands of years ago.

Successive separation and fusions of human groups suggest that racial classifications are not static.

However, the chance of finding two persons with the same total genotype discounting identical twins (Monozygotic twin) is effectively zero. Genetically each person is unique because gene is a remarkably stable chemical entity.

8 Chapter TRANSCRIPTION

DNA contains many genes for making different proteins. DNA, however, is too large a molecule to pass through the nuclear pore to go to ribosomes where proteins are prepared. DNA remains in the nucleus and through transcription; the cell makes a copy of the information in DNA which is necessary to make a particular protein. The copy is called the messenger RNA or mRNA which travels from the nucleus to the ribosomes in the cytoplasm, where the copy is used to construct a protein by means of translation.

The ingredients necessary to synthesize protein are aminoacids. Specialized molecules called transfer RNA (tRNA) carry the amino acids to ribosomes.

SEQUENCE OF EVENTS

Synthesis of proteins involves transcription– making a copy of part of information in DNA (a gene) and translation – converting that copied information into a protein.

In transcription the events to protein synthesis begin in the nucleus.

Double strands of DNA segments separate.

Each nucleotide of mRNA contains Uracil, Adenine, Cytosine or Guanine (in RNA Uracil replaces Thymine).

The number and sequence of nucleotides in DNA determine the number and sequence of nucleotides in mRNA, because DNA nucleotides only pair with specific mRNA nucleotides—as follows:

DNA Thymine with RNA's Adenine (DT-RA).

DNA Adenine with RNA's Uracil (DA-RU).

DNA Cytosine with RNA's Guanine (DC-RG).

DNA Guanine with RNA's Cytosine (DG-RC).

After the DNA nucleotides pair up RNA nucleotides, an enzyme catalyzes reaction that forms chemical bonds between RNA nucleotides to form a long mRNA segments.

Once the mRNA segments have been transcribed portions of mRNA molecule can be removed or two or more mRNA molecules can be combined.

9 Chapter TRANSLATION

The copy of DNA is called the messenger RNA or mRNA which travels from the nucleus to the ribosomes in the cytoplasm, where the copy is used to construct a protein by means of a process called translation.

It occurs in ribosomes. The mRNA molecules produced by transcription pass through nuclear pores to ribosomes. The information in mRNA is carried in groups of three nucleotides called CODONS which code for specific amino acids. There are 64 possible mRNA codons and only 20 amino acids in proteins. As a result, more than one codon can code same amino acid. Some codons do not code for amino acids but perform same functions.

Protein synthesis requires two types of RNA in addition to mRNA: tRNA and rRNA.

There is one type of tRNA for each mRNA codon. A series of three nucleotides of each tRNA molecules called "ANTICODON" pairs with codon of mRNA. Another pair of each tRNA molecule binds to a specific amino acid.

The ribosomes which consist of rRNA and proteins align mRNA with tRNA molecules, so that anticodons of tRNA pair with codons of mRNA while mRNA is attached to a ribosome.

Amino acids bound to tRNA are then joined to one another by an enzyme associated with ribosome. Enzyme causes formation of chemical bond called peptide bond, between the adjacent amino acids to form polypeptide chain consisting of many amino acids bound together by peptide bonds. The polypeptide chains then becomes folded to form a three dimensional structure of the protein molecule.

10

Chapter

MOSAICISM

It is a condition wherein there is genetically different cell type which arise from a single zygote.

Mosaicism is a very common disorder where roughly about half the population of the mammals on the earth are a type of mosaics.

The term mosaic is applied to an animal that has more than one cytogenetically distinct population of cells. For example, in human mosaic, some of the cells might be 46, XX and some 47, XXX. The fraction of cells having each genotype is quite variable, reflecting how early during embryogenesis the mosaicism originated. In most but not all cases, the mosaicism can be detected in cells from all tissues.

THE CLINICAL SIGNIFICANCE OF MOSAICISM

If the population of cytogenetically abnormal cells in a mosaic is sufficiently large, that individual will manifest disease. Conversely, if the abnormal cells are proportionally small in comparison to cytogenetically normal cells, the normal cells may be sufficient to prevent disease or prevent its severity. For example, a large majority of humans having Turner syndrome (X chromosome monosomy) die prior to birth. Many of Turner's individuals that do survive are found to be mosaics with substantial fraction of normal cells (e.g. 46XX/45XO mosaics).

X CHROMOSOME MOSAICISM

Early in embryogenesis in mammals, all but one X chromosome are functionally inactivated through a process called X chromosome inactivation. Because this inactivation occurs randomly, all normal females have roughly equal populations of two genetically different cell types and are therefore a type of mosaic. In roughly half of their cells, the paternal X chromosome has been inactivated, and in the other half the maternal X chromosome is inactive. This has a number of important biological and medical implications, particularly with regards to X linked genetic diseases.

Cats provide a unique opportunity to observe X chromosome inactivation and help visualize how it affects all females. For explanatory purpose, we will consider the orange gene (O) and its non-orange allele (o), to both be X linked. Normal male cats have a single X chromosome and can carry either the O or o gene, leading them to have an orange or black coat, respectively.

Female cats, with two X chromosomes, can have any of the three genotypes relative to the orange gene: OO (orange coat), oo (black coat) or Oo (tortoise shell or calico). The tortoise shell pattern of fine patches of black and orange reflects the pattern of X chromosome inactivation in the hair follicles.

The pattern of X chromosome inactivation seen as black and orange fur in the coat of a tortoise shell cat is present in all tissues of all female mammals. That pattern is just not usually visible because, for example, human skin colors are not encoded by X linked genes. However, understanding X chromosome inactivation and mosaicism is of great importance in all species for understanding the pathophysiology of X linked genetic diseases.

Chapter 11

CHIMERISM

Chimerism is a condition where the individual will have cell lines derived from more than one zygote.

In mythology, chimera is a fire-breathing monster, composed with a lion's head, a goat's body and serpent's tail.

In medical science a chimera is an individual having more than one genetically-distinct population of cells that originated from more than one zygote.

A chimera is something which is not likely to come across unless there is an experimental embryologist or raise cattle.

Major clinical significance is seen when one fetus is a female and one a male. In such case, the female fetus is exposed to hormones from the male and is masculinized. Such female cattle are called FREEMARTINS. The external genital tract of a freemartin looks a female, although usually infantile. The degree to which the internal genital tract is masculinized varies, but typically, the vagina is very short and uterine horns are rudimentary. Obviously, these animals are sterile. Freemartins are seen occasionally in other species, although much less commonly than in cattle, probably because those animals don't have the propensity seen in cattle to form vascular anastomoses among fetuses early in gestation.

There are reports of naturally occurring chimerism in a variety of species. Such individuals undoubtedly do occur, although they are quite rare. The most likely pathogenesis in such cases is fusion of two early embryos into one. This is suspected because chimeras are also produced experimentally, and have been a valuable research tool in several biomedical disciplines. The basic technique is to combine two very early embryos such that their cells intermix and the resulting conceptus has cells from both original embryos. This technique has been widely applied with mice and has also been applied to ruminants.

The chimeric animal called "GEEP", made by combining a 'goat' and 'sheep' embryo. The chimerism evident in the skin– big patches of skin on front and rear legs are covered with wool, representing the sheep contribution of the animal, while the majority of the remainder of the body is covered with hair, being derived from goat cells.

12 Chapter NON-DISJUNCTION

It is the improper or unequal separation of chromosomes.

During the cell division, synapsis and crossing over are necessary for proper disjunction or separation of homologous pairs of chromosomes. Whenever, chromosomal abnormalities interfere with normal pairing or crossing over, there will be increase in nondisjuction. This leads to offspring with too many or too few chromosomes. This causes aneuploidy.

In gametes, the non-disjunction can take place at meiosis I or at meiosis II.

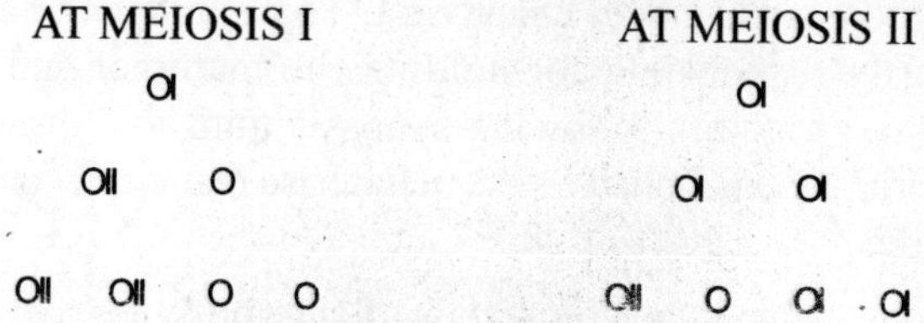

If the gamete with more number of chromosomes fertilizes with the normal opposite gamete, it leads to TRISOMY and if the gamete with less than the normal chromosomes fertilizes with the opposite normal gamete, it leads to MONOSOMY.

If non-disjunction takes place in both gametes and fertilization takes place between the cells (gametes) containing too many chromosomes, it leads to TETRASOMY. Like this various permutations and combinations are present in non-disjunction.

13 Chapter ANAPHASE LAG

Anaphase lag, delayed movement during anaphase of one homologous chromosome in mitosis or of one chromatid in meiosis, so that the chromosome is not incorporated into the nucleus of one of the daughter cells; the result is one normal cell and one cell with monosomy.

Under normal circumstances the unattached chromosome would send a signal delaying anaphase I until it is correctly tethered to a microtubule and positioned in the metaphase plane. However, lack of such a signal or a defective signal would allow anaphase to proceed before correct positioning occurred.

Recombination occurs during prophase I, and the crossover bridges connect chromosomes until anaphase I. These bridges or chiasmata are primarily responsible for holding the maternal and paternal chromosomes together following synapsis until the chromosomes are appropriately positioned on the metaphase plane and connected to microtubules.

Cohesions connect the chromatids of chromosomes together until anaphase II. The cohesions are responsible for correct orientation and microtubule tethering prior to **Meiotic Chromosome Missegregation**.

Meiosis includes a chromosome division between chromatin replication and a mitosis-like chromatid division. Several observations are important with respect to abnormal chromosome or chromatid segregation during meiosis.

1. Meiosis I errors (chromosome missegregation) tend to be more frequent than meiosis II errors (chromatid missegregation).

2. Meiosis I errors (but not meiosis II errors) exhibit a strong maternal age effect: older mothers experience conception of trisomic children more often than do younger mothers. The extra chromosome is derived from an anaphase I problem during oogenesis.

3. Mutation of the gene encoding the signal that activates the APC complex in yeast (causing the pre-anaphase checkpoint to fail) increases the frequency of meiosis I (but not meiosis II) errors.

4. Studies of women who have birthed Down syndrome infants (trisomy 21) have revealed a reduction in recombination of chromosome 21 in these women.

A human female embryo has experienced an anaphase lag event at a stage when the abnormal cells (45 chromosomes) will eventually account for 20% of *both* her somatic and germ cell populations. This error affects the individual who develops from this embryo as follows:

A. Due to the small proportion of cells involved, no effects would be observed.

B. This person would most likely appear clinically normal, but she would have an increased risk for loss of monosomic conception.

C. She would have a very high risk for uterine cancer.

D. She would most likely be unable to have children.

E. She is at high risk for birth defects.

Predict the outcome of anaphase lag, during the first mitotic division following conception, assuming this is the only chromatid attachment error. The individual in whom this error occurs would most likely to have:

1. Two cell populations, one with 46 and one with 45 chromosomes.

2. Three cell populations possessing 45, 46 or 47 chromosomes respectively.

3. One cell population with 45 chromosomes.

4. One cell population with 47 chromosomes.

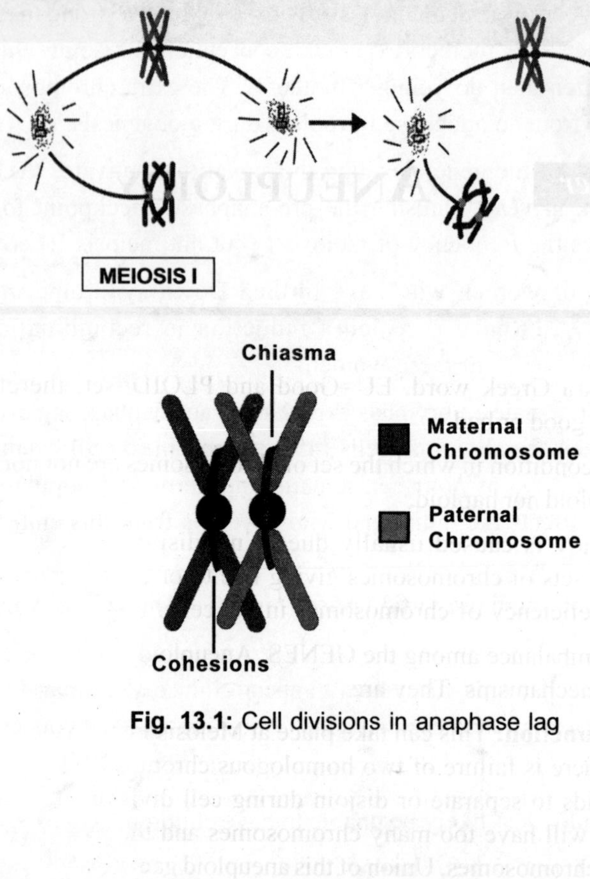

Fig. 13.1: Cell divisions in anaphase lag

14 Chapter ANEUPLOIDY

Euploidy is a Greek word, EU=Good and PLOID=set; therefore ANEU=not good or bad.

This is a condition in which the set of chromosomes are not normal –neither diploid nor haploid.

Aneuploidy is caused usually due to nondisjunction. It is the unbalanced sets of chromosomes giving rise to or consists of either excess or deficiency of chromosomes in the cells.

It is the imbalance among the GENES. Aneuploidy can arise by a variety of mechanisms. They are:

1. **Nondisjunction:** This can take place at Meiosis I or at Meiosis II. In this there is failure of two homologous chromosomes or sister chromatids to separate or disjoin during cell division. Therefore one cell will have too many chromosomes and the other cell has too less chromosomes. Union of this aneuploid gamete with euploid gamete leads to aneuploidy in the zygote.
2. **Mosaicism:** In mitotic nondisjunction however the zygote may be normal with aneuploidy occurring some time during its later development. If the resultant cells survive and continue to divide, they give rise to descendant line / descendant lines of aneuploid cells. The individual has a mixture of cells with different chromosome numbers and it is called mosaic.

   This anomaly occurs in somatic cells or in cells destined to give rise to gametes; such a case can lead to aneuploidy among offspring as well. Such a condition is called germinal mosaicism.

If the nondisjunction takes place earlier during development, the proportion of aneuploid cells found in the mosaics is larger.

If nondisjunction occurs during 1st cleavage division of zygote, then all the cells will be aneuploid. If the nondisjunction occurs at 2nd cleavage division, only half the resulting cells will be aneuploid. Half will be monosomic and half will be trisomic.

Nondisjunction in 3rd cleavage division will initially make ¼ of cells aneuploid. If the nondisjunction takes place late in development, only a tiny group of cells are aneuploid and they may escape detection. Embryos with high proportions of abnormal cells may not survive at all and they are spontaneously aborted. Mosaics can also arise from other processes.

3. The most frequent cause is the chromosome loss whereby a chromosome lags so far behind during anaphase that it is not included in either of the daughter nucleus. Consequently, one of the daughter cells will contain one less chromosome than the other (anaphase lag). If the original cell is euploid, one of the daughter cells will be monosomic.If the original cell was trisomic, and then following the loss of the extra chromosome, one daughter cell will be normal, rather than trisomic. This may lead to mosaicism.

Chromosome loss can occur at any level– either at mitosis or at meiosis and can involve autosomes or sex chromosomes.

The autosomal aneuploids are Trisomy 13, 18, 21 etc. and sex chromosomal aneuploids are Turner syndrome and Klinefelter syndrome.

Because of lionization, sex chromosomal aneuploidy is better tolerated than the autosomal aneuploidy.

Aneuploidy of large autosomes is usually lethal. Trisomies are better tolerated than monosomies.

15

Chapter

MUTATION

During the process of copying, the genes and DNA exhibit mistakes and produce abnormal genes. This process is called 'Mutation'.

DEFINITION

It is a change in DNA that may adversely affect the phenotype of an organism.

Mutations occur at random. If it occurs in one way, i.e. change from one allele to another, it produces alterations in the frequency of a particular allele in a population– it is called 'Mutation Pressure or Genetic Load'.

There are 2 types of mutations:

1. Germinal mutation.
2. Somatic mutation.

1. *Germinal mutation:* This occurs in the cells which are destined to become ova or sperms.

   This does not affect the person in whom it occurs, but it can be transmitted to and harm the future generations.

2. *Somatic mutation:* It occurs in the body cells, e.g., lungs, liver, and intestines. Not ancestral to gametes. It can affect the phenotype of the carrier but will not be transmitted to the offspring. This is involved in some steps leading to the developing of cancer.

The effect of a mutated gene on the phenotype of an organism ranges from trivial to lethal. It depends on protein properties of altered gene. The mutations that occur haphazardly, irrespective of known environmental conditions are called 'spontaneous mutations'.

Gene changes following exposure to an agent called 'mutagen' is known to produce mutation called 'induced mutation'. Mutagens include – cigarette smoke, some industrial chemicals, pesticides, various substances in waste land fills, food additives, drugs, medical and dental X-rays, ultraviolet light, radiation from past atomic tests of weapons, atomic warfare, nuclear power industry– a list that reflects on our technological society, environment and modern life styles.

Average mutation rate in human genes: It is heterogeneous. Ranges from a high of about 73 to a low of 2 mutations per million gametes per generation. Therefore an average rate is one mutation per million gamete per generation.

Sex difference in mutation: Division dependent mutation is common or greater in males because spermatogonial stem cells continue to proliferate at the rate of about 23 divisions per year. Example: Mature sperm of a 38-year-old man may have passed through 300 more divisions than mature sperm of a 25-year-old man. This age effect would not be expected in females.

Mutation can occur in any cell, at any time, but many of them probably happen at the time of DNA replication.

Mutations are: 1. Dominant 2. Recessive.

Dominant mutations are expressed in single dose irrespective of sex chromosomes or autosomes. Two are needed (male or female gamete chromosomes) for the expression of autosomal recessive traits. One mutant gene causes the expression of X-linked recessive trait in males, whereas two are needed for autosomal recessive. Sometimes mutation is reversal (reversal to normal mutation).

CLASSIFICATION OF MUTATIONS

Gene mutation	*Chromosomal mutation*	*Genomic mutation*
A. Somatic mutation	Deletion	1. Aneuploidy
B. Spontaneous mutation	Duplication	2. Monosomy
C. Induced mutation	Inversion	3. Polyploidy
D. Germinal mutation	Ring chromosome	
E. Biochemical mutation	Isochromosome	
F. Spurious mutation		
G. Reverse mutation		
H. Lethal mutation		

16 Chapter GENETIC DISORDERS

They are classified into:

1. Single gene disorders.
2. Chromosomal disorders.
3. Multifactorial disorders.
4. Mitochondrial disorders.

SINGLE GENE DISORDERS

Caused by Mutant Genes

- Single Gene Disorders
  - Autosomal
    - Dominant
      - Dentinogenesis Imperfecta, Achondroplasia
    - Recessesive
      - Cystic fibrosis
  - Sex chromosonal
    - X linked disorder
      - Dominant
        - Hyperphosphatemia OR (Vit. D Resistant Rickets)
      - Recessive
        - Hemophilia

Fragile X chromosome is both dominant and recessive.

Y chromosomal disorders are called holandric disorders.

- Mutations are present on one chromosome of any given pair or on both chromosomes of that pair.
- Cause of the defect is single major error in genetic information.
- Exhibit obvious and characteristic pedigree patterns.
- Frequency is 1 in 2000.
- Single gene disorders are classified as follows:

CHROMOSOMAL DISORDERS

a. The defect arises from an 'excess' or 'deficiency' of whole chromosome.

b. As a group, the chromosome disorders are common.

c. The incidence is 7 per 1000 live births.

d. Account for about half of all spontaneous, first trimester abortions.

The chromosomal disorders can be **structural** abnormalities **OR numerical** abnormalities.

In **structural** abnormalities there can be:

A. Reciprocal translocation

B. Deletion

C. Ring chromosome

D. Duplication

E. Inversion

F. Isochromosome.

G. Robertsonian translocation.

In **numerical** abnormalities, there can be:

1. Aneuploidy.
2. Polyploidy.

Aneuploidy is the increase or decrease in any of the pairs of chromosomes in a particular group (from A to G).

It can be thus:

(a) Monosomy (b) Trisomy (c) Polysomy

In polyploidy there is increase in the haploid number of chromosomes– three times, four times or more (multiples of haploid number).

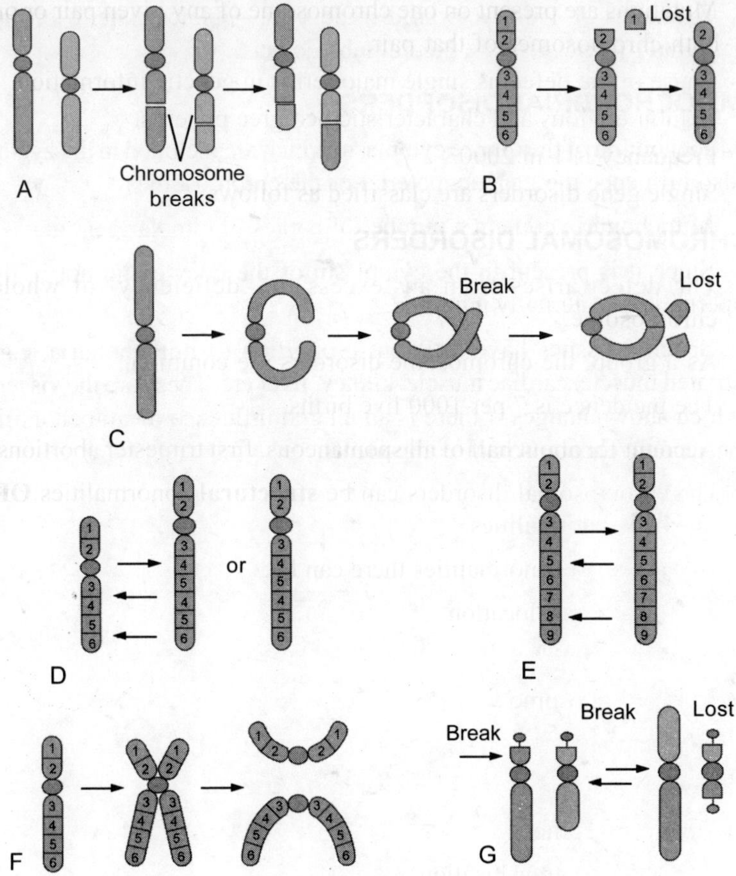

Fig. 16.1: Structural abnormalities of chromosomes

That can be 23X3, 23X4 and so on.

MULTIFACTORIAL DISORDERS

a. Are associated with multiple disorders resulting from genetic and environmental factors.

b. The environmental cause can be either infection or teratogen.

c. Tend to recur in families but do not show characteristic pedigree patterns of single gene traits.

d. May affect more than one member of the family at a time.

Examples of Multifactorial disorders are – Cleft palate, Cleft lip, Familial pyloric stenosis, Neural tube defects.

MITOCHONDRIAL DISORDERS

Mitochondria of the oocyte cytoplasm which are included in the zygote also influence the genetic material or the chromosomes.

Mitochondria contain a number of copies of circular genome.

Since it is present in the cytoplasm of the oocyte and not in the sperm, it is maternally inherited.

Specific tissues have different proportion of mitochondria, e.g., striated muscle, cardiac muscle, kidney, liver etc. These are the viscera which show changes if there is an altered influence of mitochondria on genetic/chromosomal components.

17 Chapter

CHROMOSOMAL DISORDERS

STRUCTURAL DISORDERS

Wolf Hirshhorn Syndrome

Also called 4p – syndrome.

In this disorder there is deletion of 'p' arm of 4th pair of chromosomes – one or both in 4th pair.

Karyotyping: 46, XX 4p- OR 46, XY 4p-.

Features:

1. Improper fusion in the midline of the body
2. Wide set eyes.
3. Broad nose.
4. Low set, malformed ears.
5. Small lower jaw.
6. Cleft palate.
7. Heart, lungs and skeletal abnormalities.
8. Improperly fused penis.
9. Low birth weight.

These fetuses or newborns fail to thrive and die young.

Cri Du Chat Syndrome or Cat Cry Syndrome

This condition is caused due to complete or partial deletion of short arm of chromosome 5. The newborns with 5p– usually have high pitched mewing cry like that of a kitten, therefore it is called Cat Cry Syndrome.

Incidence: One in 50,000 live births.

Karyotyping: 46, XX 5p- or 46, XY 5p-.

Features:

1. Moon face with wide set eyes in newborns.
2. Epicanthic folds persistent on upper eye lids.
3. Malformed and low set ears.
4. Small head.
5. Slow growth.
6. Mental retardation.
7. High pitched mewing cry like that of a kitten.

Prader-Willi Syndrome

This is a condition where there are tiny deletions of 15 q near centromere.

Karyotyping: 46, XX, 15q- or 46, XY, 15q-.

Features:

1. Poor muscle tone.
2. Poor reflexes.
3. Poor feeding.
4. Mental retardation.
5. Extremely obese.
6. Short stature with small hands and feet.
7. Under developed gonads and external genitalia.

NUMERICAL DISORDERS

Trisomy

This occurs due to anaphase lag which causes nondisjunction and one cell gets excess chromosomes. The trisomies of all the sets of chromosomes are noted but very few grow up to full term and some survive after the birth.

The following are the most common trisomic disorders which have been observed in autosomes.

Trisomy 13 (Patau Syndrome)

This was identified in 1960 by Patau and associates, therefore termed 'Patau syndrome'.

It is an autosomal trisomy of 13th chromosome.

Karyotyping: 47 XX/XY + 13.

It is a severe disorder, lethal in about half the live born infants within first month.

Cause: Nondisjunction and in about 20% of cases caused by translocation.

Features:

1. Severe central nervous system malformations leading to mental retardation, arhinencephaly, holoprosencephaly.
2. Growth retardation.
3. Sloping forehead.
4. Ocular hypertelorism.
5. Microphthalmia.
6. Iris coloboma or absence of eyes.
7. Malformed ears.
8. Hare lip.
9. Cleft palate.
10. Post axial polydactily in hands and feet.
11. Clenched hands with 1st and 5th digits overlapping 3rd and 4th digits.
12. Rocker bottom feet due to prominent calcanei.
13. Simian crease sometimes present.
14. Congenital heart defects.
15. Congenital urogenital defects.
16. Cryptorchidism in male; bicornuate uterus in female along with hypoplastic ovaries.

Trisomy 18 or Edward Syndrome

Described by Edward and colleagues in 1960, therefore the name.

It is an autosomal disorder.

Trisomy of 18th chromosome occurs in this case.

Incidence: One in 8000 newborns. About 95% of Trisomy 18 fetuses abort spontaneously.

Postnatal survival in 10% of cases upto one year.

The age limit, upper and lower, is 2 months to 15 years. 80% of the patients are females.

This is due to advanced maternal age because of nondisjunction.

Karyotyping: 47, XX or XY + 18.

Features:

1. Severe growth retardation.
2. Mental retardation.
3. Craniofacial dysmorphism.– head has prominent occiput, thus it is elongated.
4. The jaw recedes and is called micrognathia.
5. Hare lip.
6. Low set ears.
7. Short neck.
8. Rocker bottom deformity of feet due to prominent calcaneii.
9. Tightly clenched fists with 2nd and 5th digits overlapping 3rd and 4th digits.
10. Genital abnormalities.
11. Severe congenital abnormalities of heart, alimentary canal, renal system and respiratory system.
12. Short sternum.
13. Simian crease may be present.
14. Hypoplastic thick nails.

Trisomy 21 or Down Syndrome or Mongolism

First described by Langdon Down in 1866.

This is caused due to late maternal age (elderly primi/above 35 years).

There is a peculiar pattern within families.

Incidence: One in 800.

Is an autosomal disorder.

The extra chromosome is the small acrocentric chromosome 21.

It is due to nondisjunction in male than in female (paternal nondisjunction).

In both sexes the incident or accident is more likely to happen at meiosis I.

It is called Mongolism due to the presence of characteristic epicanthic folds which give a slanting appearance to the eyes. It is diagnosed at birth or shortly after birth.

Features:

1. Oblique palpebral fissures.
2. Epicanthic folds.
3. Flat occiput.
4. Broad and short neck.
5. Short and broad hands.
6. Short fingers and clinodactyly with incurving of 5th finger.
7. Excessive space between the first and second toes, furrow extending proximally along the plantar base of the toes and sole.
8. Presence of Simian crease at the bases of medial four fingers.
9. Habitually open mouth due to large tongue.
10. Tongue is not only large, it also has furrows and lacks central fissure.
11. Small genitalia.
12. Muscular hypotonia.
13. Mental retardation.
14. Usually associated with Klinefelter syndrome.
15. There will be increased risk of leukemia.
16. One third of patients have congenital malformations of the heart.

17. Radiographically, acetabular and iliac angles are decreased.
18. Premature senility associated with cortical atrophy.
19. Ventricular dilatation and neurolfibrillar tangles.

Translocation Down Syndrome

In about 4% of people with Down syndrome have 46 rather than 47 chromosomes, one of which is abnormally long. This long chromosome is a Robertsonian translocation, usually involving chromosomes 14 and 21. Because nondisjunction is not the cause, no maternal age effect is seen here. These kinds of cases are very few but recur in the same family.

A carrier parent of an individual with translocation Down syndrome may have only 45 chromosomes, one of which is 14q21q. Three chromosomes in this translocation heterozygote contain nearly all of the material present in original four chromosomes. The tiny tips of chromosomes 14 and 21 are lost, but in this carrier is unaffected (no essential genetic materials are missing).

During meiosis, two chromosomes will usually proceed to one pole and one to the other pole, thus six types of gametes are possible; of these two are balanced – one bearing the normal chromosomes 14 and 21 and another carrying single large 14q21q translocation. When combined with structurally normal chromosomes during fertilization, the former will yield a normal zygote and latter give rise to a translocation heterozygote with a normal phenotype. Thus a translocation may pass unnoticed through a number of generations. Among the types of unbalanced gametes produced by a carrier, only one will lead to a viable zygote after combining with a gamete with normal chromosomes. This zygote will have an extra dose of chromosome 21 and will develop Down syndrome.

A carrier parent may therefore produce up to three kinds of offspring:

1. Phenotypically, karyotypically normal.
2. Phenotypically unaffected translocation heterozygote.
3. Translocation Down syndrome.

The theoretical risk of having a child with Down syndrome is thus 1/3 but actual observed frequencies show considerable variation.

SEX CHROMOSOMAL DISORDERS

Trisomies / Polysomies

Klinefelter Syndrome

This was described by Henry Klinefelter in 1942.

It is a sex chromosomal trisomy.

It is a male disorder. Along with XY, the cells present Barr body.

This disorder is recognized only after puberty or accidentally if the epithelial cells are examined for some other reasons, or if the chromosome study is done routinely before puberty.

It is due to nondisjunction in gonadal cells– in oocytes sperms, either at meiosis I or meiosis II.

Features:

1. Tall and eunuchoid with legs longer in proportion.
2. Weight is above normal.
3. Head circumference is small at birth.
4. Secondary sexual characters are poorly developed.
5. Small testes.
6. Hyalinization of seminiferous tubules therefore sterile.
7. Verbal I.Q. is less.
8. High incidence of educational problems.
9. Less aggressive and less active.
10. More susceptible to social stress.

Triple - X Syndrome (XXX Syndrome)

- Also called Poly X females.
- This disorder was first reported in 1959.
- There is no specific phenotype except that there is tendency to be tall and thin.
- Frequency/Incidence: One in 10,000 newborns.
- Individual is always female. Appear completely normal.

  There may be:
- Mental retardation.

- Psychosis.
- Educational and behavioral problems.
- Menstrual disorders but fertile.

Karyotyping: 47, XXX: 48, XXXX, 49, XXXXX etc.

Cause:

a. Nondisjunction– in case of more than three X chromosomes the nondisjunction is associated with both gametes. In females (mother) nondisjunction is in meiosis I.

b. Late maternal age.

c. Mosaicism.

Monosomy

Autosomal monosomies are lethal. Sex chromosomal monosomy is noted in females and is called Turner syndrome.

Turner Syndrome

- Described in 1938 by Turner.
- This is a sex chromosomal monosomy.
- It is a disorder seen in females.
- Karyotyping: 45, XO.
- There is lack of one X chromosome.

Features:

1. Sexual infantilism.
2. Short stature.
3. Cubitus valgus (reduced/prominent carrying angle).
4. Webbing of the neck.
5. Low hair line at the nape.
6. Characteristic facial appearance.
7. Wide chest.
8. Broadly spaced nipples.
9. Lymphedema of the feet.
10. External genitalia are juvenile.

11. Axillary and pubic hairs are sparse.
12. Intelligence is normal or slightly reduced.

On Examination:

a. Dematoglyphics unusual with high total ridge count.
b. Coarctation of aorta.
c. Congenital heart disorders.
d. Internal sexual organs are female.
e. Ovaries are streak like only connective tissue is present.
f. The ovarian stroma and ovarian follicles may be present prenatally but absent postnatally.
g. Have defective spatial perception.

18 Chapter

FRAGILE X-SYNDROME

This is a condition where a fragile site is present in band q27.3 of X chromosome roughly in 1250 males in upto 50% of his tested cells.

There are about 20 different heritable fragile sites existing on other chromosomes but none of them is associated with any particular phenotype.

It was in 1969, when this disorder was identified. The defect was noticed as a constriction in the long arm of X chromosome in mentally retarded males. This cytological defect is associated with chromosome breakage; it was called FRAGILE X-SYNDROME. Most of the males are moderately to severely mentally retarded. The condition is associated with huge testes, large, protruding ears, long jaw, big head, stubby hands, lax joints, heart valve defect, tall as children but short as adults. Speech is delayed in development and high pitched, repetitive in nature and jocular. Sometimes hyperactive/autistic as children but in teenage and adulthood they are shy and nonassertive but friendly. Few are fertile.

In females– One in 2250 are affected roughly.

Affected females are mildly to moderately mentally retarded. A kind of learning disability but no consistent physical abnormalities. Females are usually the carriers. Fragile X carriers are highly fertile and frequency of twins is more.

19

Chapter

TESTICULAR FEMINISATION

It is an X linked recessive trait occurring in individuals who are chromosomally male (46, XY).

The gene is located on the long arm of X chromosome near the centromere. The affected individuals produce plenty of male hormones but the receptors of androgens are absent or defective, therefore unable to respond to hormone's masculanising effect. Therefore affected individuals develop as phenotypic females.

Frequency: 1 in 65,000 46, XY individuals. This condition is also called ANDROGEN INSTABILITY SYNDROME.

Features:

1. Tall stature.
2. Face is feminine without any trace of hair on the face.
3. No pubic or Axillary hair.
4. Well developed breasts.
5. Normal vulva.
6. Vagina ends in a blind pouch-depth is 8 to 20 cms.
7. Absence of female internal reproductive organs.
8. Absence of menstruation.
9. They are sterile.
10. Male genotypically but female from the psychosocial aspect.

20 Chapter TRANSLOCATION

Break in two or more non homologous chromosomes, followed by reattachments in new combinations, can lead to formations of translocations.

Definition: It is the transfer of genetic material from one chromosome to another.

There are two types of translocations. They are:

1. Reciprocal translocation.
2. Robertsonian translocation.

RECIPROCAL TRANSLOCATION

Occurs when two different chromosomes exchange segments. In this the rearrangement of chromosome parts is complete with no left-over pieces. Because all of the genetic material is still present but in a different arrangement a heterozygote for such translocation is said to be 'balanced'. Rate of such translocation is 1 in 500 persons. A break occurs in each chromosome and the segments below the break switch positions.

In 'unbalanced' type the egg or the sperm have either extra chromosomal material or not enough chromosomal material.

ROBERTSONIAN TRANSLOCATION

Occurs when two chromosomes join around their centers. Translocations between and among acrocentric chromosomes i.e., between 13, 14, 15 (D group) and 21, 22 (G group).

The long arms of two acrocentric chromosomes are joined together at the centromere, as are the two heterochromatic tips. The tiny heterochromatic chromosomes so formed, which apparently carry no important genes, is usually lost. But the longer translocated chromosome contains the full compliment of essential genes from two nonhomologous chromosomes. The gamete with this balanced chromosome when combined with a normal gamete, gives rise to a balanced heterozygote. The resulting individual has total of 45 chromosomes but phenotypically normal.

Another type of aberration is a metacentric chromosome consisting of two identical arms. This may or may not represent an actual translocation. Such chromosomes are called 'Isochromosome' and are thought to be formed by misdivision of centromeres (Instead of lengthwise division there will be cross wise division between duplicate chromatids), thereby joining two identical chromatid arms. Union of broken sister chromatid arms also can produce isochromosome. During meiosis, 2 isochromosomes separate, 50% of gametes contain a duplication of one arm and deletion of the other.

Isochromosomes for long arm of group D or G chromosomes, when heterozygous with normal chromosomes, lead to effective trisomy for that chromosome even though the total number of chromosome is only 46. Few cases of Down syndrome are known to have a long arm isochromosome of 21 and a normal chromosome.

21 Chapter PEDIGREE

Meaning– A line of ancestors of known descent.

DEFINITION

It is a record of inheritance of certain genetic traits for two or more generations presented in the form of diagram or family tree.

It is summarization of information about the family in a diagrammatic form.

The symbols used in preparing the pedigree chart are internationally accepted.

It is useful for genetic counsellors to advise intending couple about the possibilities of having children with genetic defects.

The person through the pedigree chart is prepared is called PROBAND or PROPOSITUS. Proband is indicated by an arrow.

The Pedigree Preparation

1. Each generation occupies a separate horizontal line.
2. Most ancestral at the top and are numbered from top to bottom by Roman numerals.
3. Individuals within a given generation (sibs) are numbered from left to right and numbered in Arabic numerals.
4. Arranged according to birth order – eldest to youngest– from left to right.
5. Unshaded symbols–normal. Shaded symbols–diseased or dead and half shaded–dominant disorder.

Difficulties in Getting Information

1. Very few people keep careful written records of the family
2. Recollections may be hazy or exaggerated especially about medical history.
3. Abortions, artificial insemination, adoptation and illegitimate births may go unnoticed or unmentioned.
4. Number of abortions and gestational age at the time of abortions, sex of the aborted fetus or the still born is usually lacking while recollecting the information.
5. There may be reluctance to discuss about the members of the family who are in some way abnormal.
6. Close relatives may be unaware of the members of the family who died young or institutionised for the disease.
7. Phenotype expression of a trait often varies among individuals specially when there is autosomal recessive disease.

SYMBOLS USED

Normal female	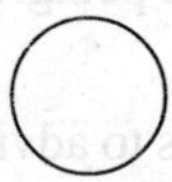	Diseased male	
Normal male	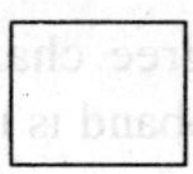	Affected female	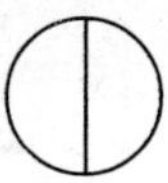
Sex not specified	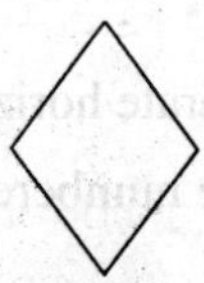	Affected male	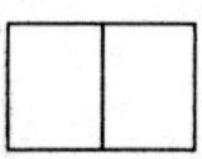
Miscarriage	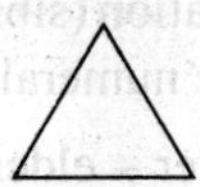	Carrier female	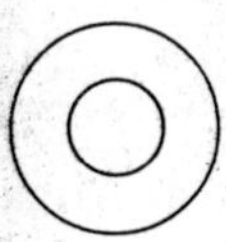
Diseased female		Carrier male	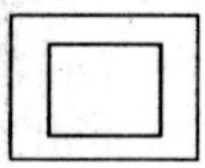

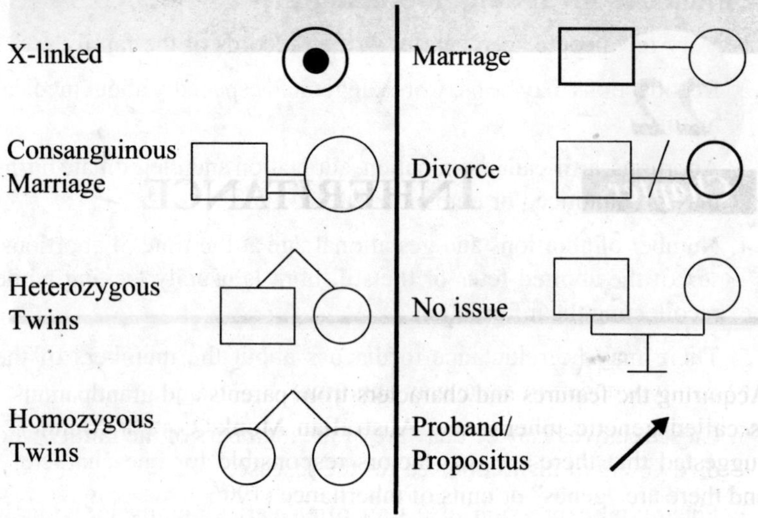
X-linked
Marriage
Consanguinous
Marriage
Divorce
Heterozygous
Twins
No issue
Homozygous
Twins
Proband/
Propositus

22 Chapter INHERITANCE

Acquiring the features and characters from parents and grandparents is called genetic inheritance. Australian Monk, Gregor Mendel, suggested that there are two factors responsible for one character and there are "genes" or units of inheritance (1906).The character of parents as a "unit" may not appear in first generation but may appear quite unchanged in later generations.

Genetic inheritance is classified into:

1. Autosomal.
2. Sex chromosomal.

Autosomal inheritance is further classified into:

i. Autosomal dominant.
ii. Autosomal recessive.

Sex chromosomal inheritance can be further classified into:

i. X-linked.
ii. Y- linked (Holandric).

X- linked can be classified into:

i. Dominant.
ii. Recessive.

Almost all disorders caused by defects in non-enzymic or structural proteins are often inherited as dominant disorders; and disorders caused by enzyme deficiencies are recessive inheritance.

To determine the inheritance of the disorder, pedigree is a must.

But some pedigrees for X linked recessive inheritance also fit into an autosomal gene acting as a dominant inheritance in males and recessive inheritance in females. Therefore it is necessary to pool together many studies and analyze the data.

Sometimes mutations at different loci may occasionally give rise to very similar phenotypes. Some inherited disorders do have multiple modes of transmission.

AUTOSOMAL DOMINANT INHERITANCE

1. All affected individuals have at least one affected parent.
2. Affected individuals are usually found in every generation of a sizable pedigree that is there is no skipping generations.
3. Both males and females are affected in equal number.
4. Males and females transmit the trait–male to male transsmission rules out X linkage and female to female transmission rules out Y linkage.
5. Mating of heterozygous affected with unaffected individuals produce about half affected and half unaffected offspring or on an average the trait is transmitted by an affected parent to half of the children born.
6. The trait does not appear in the descendants of two unaffected parents unless the dominant allele is reintroduced by mating with unrelated affected individuals.
7. The trait may be more severe or extreme in homozygotes than in hetero zygotes or it may even be lethal.
8. The sex of the child born is not influenced by the transmission or occurrence of the trait.

   The most common autosomal dominant traits are:

   I. Dentinogenesis imperfecta.
   II. Achondroplasia.
   III. Familial hyper cholesterolemia.
   IV. Huntington's disease.

AUTOSOMAL RECESSIVE INHERITANCE

This trait appears only in sibs and not in parents who are carriers

1. The most affected individuals have two unaffected parents (two carriers produce an affected child).
2. The trait is expressed in both sexes and transmitted by either sex to both male and female offspring in roughly equal numbers.
3. Mating between unaffected heterozygotes yield about ¾ unaffected and ¼ affected off spring or the risk of recurrence is 1:4.
4. With the rare traits the unaffected but heterozygous parents of an affected individual may be related to each other.
5. Mating between an affected and unaffected parents will usually yield all unaffected off spring.
6. When both parents are affected all their children are affected.
7. Autosomal recessive traits often do not appear in every generation.
8. There is consanguineous marriage between the parents of the affected individual.

Examples:

1. Cystic fibrosis.
2. Albinism.
3. Glycogen storage disease.
4. Retinitis pigmentosa.

X LINKED DOMINANT INHERITANCE

It is relatively rare because when families are small it may be impossible to distinguish X linked dominant from autosomal dominant inheritance. Only few disorders are known.

1. There is no male to male transmission of the trait.
2. Affected males mate unaffected females they produce all unaffected sons and all affected daughters.
3. Affected females can produce affected sons and daughters as well as unaffected sons and daughters. Among these ratio of sons and daughters of affected to unaffected is 1:1.
4. Every affected individual has one affected parent but affected for males the affected parent is always the mother.

5. Males being homozygous are usually more severely affected than females who are heterozygous.
6. Owing to the phenomenon of X-chromosome inactivation expression of trait is also more variable among females.
7. If affected males and affected females reproduce at the same rate in the population as a whole there will be twice as many affected males and females. This is because males have one X-chromosome where females have two X-chromosomes.

Example: Hypophosphatemia or Vitamin D resistant rickets.

X LINKED RECESSIVE INHERITANCE

1. Males are usually showing the trait, being uncommon in females.
2. The traits will pass from father through his daughters and to all his grand-sons.
3. The trait requires series of carrier females for transmission to males and thus the affected males are related to each other through females.

Example: Hemophilia.

Y LINKED INHERITANCE

It is called holandric inheritance. Only three to four loci have been definitely assigned to the Y-chromosome. Besides these some factors for sperm production, skeletal height and tooth size have been provisionally assigned to the Y-chromosome.

Female descendents lacking nonhomogenous Y-region could neither receive, express nor transmit such a trait.

The traits of non homologous genes present on Y-chromosome are always seen only in males. Affected males transmit trait to all his sons and none to daughters. All the genes present on Y-chromosome are always expressed phenotypically as there is no homologous Y-chromosome but X-chromosome will have homologous and non-homologous regions.

FACTORS LEADING TO VARIATION IN EXPRESSION OF GENES

1. **Penetrance:** It is the ability of the gene to express phenotypically and inability is called as nonpenetrance.

2. **Expressivity:** Phenotypic expression of an abnormal trait may not be of the same degree in all the individuals having that gene. This expression is between two extremities/extremes– normal and abnormal.
3. **Pleiotropy:** When a single gene is responsible for a number of distinct and unrelated phenotypic traits, leading to one gene several effects. Thus many genetic defects forming a syndrome are examples of pleiotropy.
4. **Association linkage:** Non-random occurrence of two phenotypically separate traits in a population, e.g., trait for blood group 'O' and peptic ulcer and duodenum show a significant association. When the genes for two different traits are situated close to each other on the same chromosomes, there are greater chances that the two genes will be transmitted together, contradicting the Mendel's law of independent assortment which has been found to be true only when the genes under study are found to be situated on two different chromosomes.

23 Chapter PRENATAL DIAGNOSIS

This is very important and essential investigation for the genetic counselling.

It is the diagnosis of the disorders, if any, during the intrauterine life of humans.

There are two basic approaches for identifying the foetal defects.

1. Visualization of foetus.
2. Analysis of foetal tissues.

1. *Visualization of foetus is done by:*

A. **Non-invasive** method

i. Ultrasound

ii. Radiography

B. **Invasive** method

Foetoscopy.

2. *Analysis of foetal tissues:*

A. Amniocentesis.

B. Chorionic villi sampling.

C. Foetal and maternal blood analysis.

D. Foetal skin biopsy.

E. Foetal liver biopsy.

F. Foetal lung, kidney and muscle biopsy.

G. Cord blood sampling.

H. Preimplantation.

NONINVASIVE METHODS

Ultra Sonography

1. It helps in visualizing embryo of 5½ to 6 weeks.
2. Detection of cardiac activity at 7 to 8 weeks.
3. It is a routine procedure for verification of viable embryo. Major internal organs 16 to 20 weeks.
4. Determination of gestational age.
5. Diagnosis of multiple gestations, if any.
6. Determination of placental and foetal positions.
7. Diagnosis of foetal abnormalities.
8. Determination of uterine abnormalities.
9. Guides (helps) in passing the instruments for invasive procedures.
10. Detection of amniotic fluid. This is a noninvasive procedure. It is harmless to both mother and foetus. High frequency sound waves are utilized to produce visible images from the pattern of the echos made by different tissues and organs, including the baby in the amniotic cavity.

Limitations of the Procedure:

1. Subtle abnormalities may not be detected until late in pregnancy.
2. It is difficult to detect Down syndrome in early pregnancy.

Radiography

Standard anteroposterior and lateral radiographic views are essential for analysis of the foetal skeleton.

Useful for comparison with prenatal ultrasound.

Help to define anomalies when autopsy consent is limited/help to determine sites to be examined microscopically.

Conditions diagnosed by postmortem radiography. This may include:

a. Skeletal anomalies (Dwarfism, dysplasia, sinenomelia).
b. Neural tube defects (anencephaly, spina bifida).

c. Osteogenesis imperfecta (osteopenea, fractures).

d. Soft tissue changes (hydrops, hygromas).

e. Teratomas and other neoplasm.

f. Growth retardation.

g. Orientation and audit of foetal parts.

h. Assessment of catheter or therapeutic device placement.

INVASIVE METHODS

Foetoscopy

In this procedure, cannulation of umbilical vessels is done for sampling, transfusion and foetal tissues biopsy.

Amniocentesis

This is an invasive procedure. Needle of 3½", 20 gauge is passed through the mother's lower abdomen into amniotic cavity inside the uterus. Enough amniotic fluid is present for this to be accomplished. Starting about 14 weeks gestation. Between 14-20 weeks is the best period. About 20-30 ml of fluid is aspirated. Sex determination is 99% accurate. Fragile X-chromosome detected if any. Chromosome instability syndrome has been predetermined by this method. The amniotic fluid contains foetal cells mostly derived from foetal skin. These cells can be grown in culture for chromosome analysis, biochemical analysis and molecular biological analysis.

In third trimester of pregnancy the amniotic fluid can be analyzed for determination of foetal lung maturity. This is important when foetus is below 35-36 of weeks gestation. Because the lungs may not be mature enough to sustain the life. This is because lungs are not producing enough surfactant. After birth the infant will develop respiratory distress syndrome from hyaline membrane disease.

The amniotic fluid can be analyzed by fluorescence polarization (FPOL), for lecithin-sphingomyelin ratio (L: S ratio) and phosphatidyl glycerol (PG).

Risks with amniocentesis are not common. They are:

1. Foetal loss– 0.5%.

2. Maternal Rh sensitization.
3. Cannot be drawn if oligohydramnios.
4. Contamination of fluid can occur (amnionitis). If Rh sensivity is there, then Rh –ve mothers can be treated with RhoGam. If oligohydramnios is present, instillation of saline into amniotic cavity and then remove fluid for analysis.

Indications:

1. Advanced maternal age.
2. Previous child with genetic abnormality.
3. First degree relative with neural tube defect.

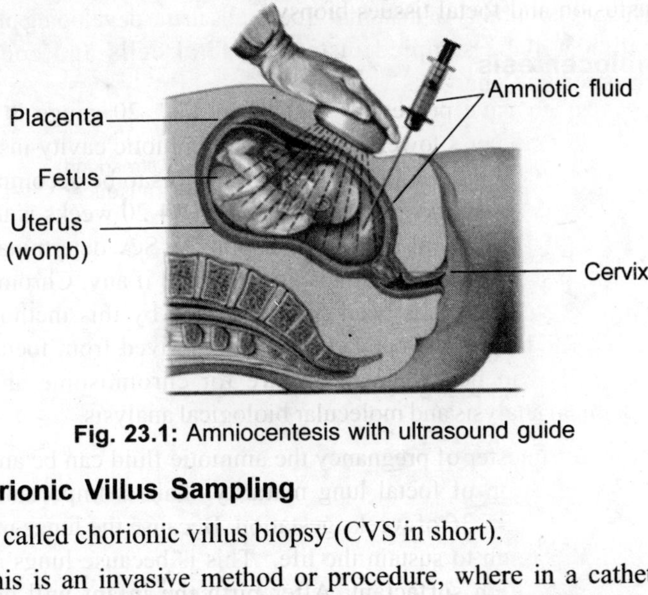

Fig. 23.1: Amniocentesis with ultrasound guide

Chorionic Villus Sampling

Also called chorionic villus biopsy (CVS in short).

This is an invasive method or procedure, where in a catheter is passed via vagina, through cervix and into the uterus to the developing placenta under the ultrasound guidance. This is called **transcervical** approach.

Alternative approaches are: **Transvaginal** and **transabdominal**.

The introduction of the catheter allows sampling of cells from the placental chorionic villi. These cells can be analyzed by a variety of techniques.

The most common test employed on the cells obtained by CVS is, chromosome analysis to determine the karyotype of the fetus.

Cells can be grown in culture for the biochemical or molecular biologic analysis.

CVS can be safely performed between 9 and 12 weeks gestation.

Disadvantage:

1. It is an invasive procedure.
2. Small but significant rate of morbidity of fetus, the loss rate is 0.5% higher than amniocentesis.
3. Possibility of maternal Rh sensitization is present.
4. There is possibility of maternal blood cells in the developing placenta which will be sampled instead of fetal cells and confound chromosome analysis.

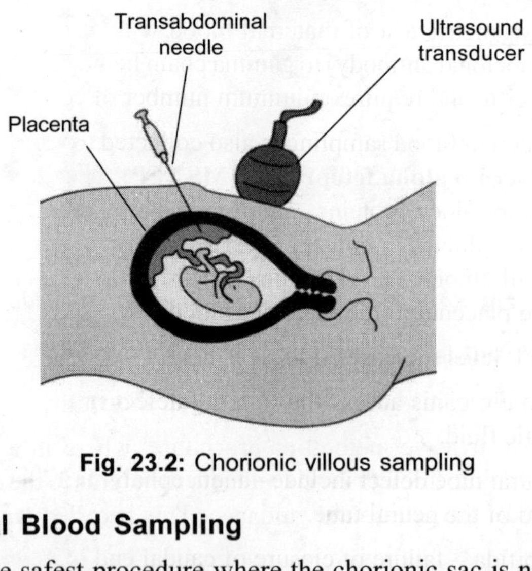

Fig. 23.2: Chorionic villous sampling

Maternal Blood Sampling

This is the safest procedure where the chorionic sac is not invaded.

This is a new technique that makes use of the phenomenon of **fetal blood cells** gaining access to maternal blood circulation through the placental villi.

Ordinarily very small amount of fetal cells enter the maternal circulation in this fashion. About 20 ml sample of maternal peripheral blood has 0-20 cells of the fetus, i.e., one fetal cell per million maternal cells.

The fetal cells can be sorted out and analyzed by variety of techniques to look for particular DNA sequences. Fluorescence in situ hybridization (FISH) is one technique that can be applied to identify particular chromosomes of the fetal cells recovered from the maternal blood and diagnose aneuploid conditions such as the trisomies and monosomy.

Disadvantage:

It is difficult to get many fetal blood cells which may not be enough to reliably determine anomalies of the fetal karyotype or assay for other abnormalities.

The fetal cells are present in maternal blood as early as 33 days of gestation. By 15 weeks they are definitely present.

Flow cytometric test of maternal blood with antigamma globulin MAb (monoclonal antibody) to gamma chain hemoglobin molecule is highly specific and requires minimum number of cells.

The maternal blood sampling is also collected to study the level of **maternal serum alpha fetoprotein (MSAFP).** The developing fetus has two major blood proteins– albumin and alpha fetoprotein (AFP). The test is conducted to note the level of AFP from the fetus. Usually only a small amount of AFP gains access to the amniotic fluid and crosses the placenta to the maternal blood.

The AFP level increases if there is neural tube defect in the fetus.

The protein gains access through the defect in the neural tube to the amniotic fluid.

The neural tube defect include– anencephaly–failure of closure of cranial end of the neural tube.

Spina bifida – failure of closure of caudal end of neural tube.

The other conditions where there is gap/defect in the anterior abdominal wall, fetal AFP increases in maternal blood, e.g. Omphalocele or Gastroschisis.

While finding out the levels of AFP in maternal serum it is important to note the gestational age because the amount of MSAFP increases with gestational age.

The race of mother and gestational diabetes are also important to know because the MSAFP can be affected by these factors. MSAFP is typically reported as multiples of the mean (MOM) – the greater the MOM, the more likely a defect is present. The MSAFP has the greatest Sensitivity between 16 and 18 weeks and useful between 15 and 22 weeks.

Disadvantages:

MSAFP can be elevated for a variety of reasons which are not related to fetal neural tube defects or abdominal wall defects. Therefore this test is not 100% specific. The most common cause for an elevated MSAFP is a wrong estimation of gestational age of the fetus. Therefore combination of MSAFP, screening and ultrasonography has to be done in suspected cases.

Neural tube defects can be distinguished from other defects by use of acetyl cholinesterase test. It is performed on amniotic fluid obtained by amniocentesis. If acetylcholinestarase is elevated along with MSAFP– then neural tube defect is likely. If acetyl cholinesterase is not detectable, then some other fetal defect is suggested.

The MSAFP level tends to be lower when Down syndrome or other chromosomal abnormalities is present.

The genetic polymorphisms due to mutations in the methylene tetrahydrofolate reductase gene may increase the risk for neural tube defects. Folate is the co-factor for this enzyme, which is part of the pathway of homocysteine metabolism in cells.

The C6 77T and A1298C mutations are associated with elevated maternal homocysteine concentrations and an increased risk for neural tube defects in fetuses. Prevention of many neural tube defects can be accomplished by supplementation of the maternal diet with only 4 mg of folic acid per day, but this vitamin supplement must be taken a month before conception and through the first trimester.

Maternal serum beta HCG: This test is used as a test for confirmation of pregnancy. Beginning at about a week following conception and implantation of the developing embryo in the uterus, the trophoblast will produce enough, detectable beta HCG to diagnose pregnancy. Thus, by the time the 1st menstrual period is missed, the beta HCG will virtually always be elevated enough to provide a positive pregnancy test. The beta HCG can also be quantified in serum from maternal blood and this can be useful early in pregnancy when threatened abortion or ectopic pregnancy is suspected, because the amount of beta HCG will be lower than expected in these conditions.

Later in pregnancy, in the middle to late second trimester, the beta HCG can be used in conjunction with the MSAFP to screen for chromosomal abnormalities– Down syndrome in particular. An elevated beta HCG coupled with a decreased MSAFP suggests Down syndrome.

Very high levels of HCG suggest trophoblastic disease (molar pregnancy). Absence of fetus on ultrasonography along with an elevated HCG suggests Hydatidiform mole or Vesicular mole.

The HCG level can be used to follow up treatment for molar pregnancy to make sure that no trophoblastic disease, such as choriocarcinoma persists.

Maternal serum estriol: The amount of estriol in the maternal blood /serum is dependent upon viable fetus, a properly functioning placenta and maternal well being. The substrate for estriol begins as dehydroepiandrosterone (DHEA) made by the fetal adrenal glands. This is further metabolized in the placenta to estriol. The estriol crosses to the maternal circulation and is excreted by the maternal kidney in urine or by the maternal liver in the bile. The measurement of serial estriol levels in the third trimester will give an indication of general well being of the fetus. If the estriol level drops, then the fetus is threatened and delivery may be necessary emergently. Estriol tends to be lower when Down syndrome is present and when there is adrenal hypoplasia with anencephaly.

Urine of the pregnant mother can be analyzed for **enzyme assay of fetal Homocysteinuria, Phenylketonuria** etc.

Fetal skin biopsy and fetal liver biopsy and various other organs like fetal lung, muscle and kidney biopsy are for Karyotyping. Speciman must be fresh and without contamination. For that, the tissue samples are washed in sterile saline prior to placing them in culture media.

Placenta, lung, diaphragm undergo least maceration therefore they are preferred. Obtaining tissue from more than one site can increase the yield by avoiding contamination, or detection of mosaicism.

The cells of the above mentioned organs are not only used for karyotyping, they are also used for FISH technique, DNA analysis and probes. PCR technique can be applied for diagnosis. These methods help in minority of cases.

Microbiologic culture of tissues obtained are tested for congenital infections which include– TORCH.

T- Toxoplasmosis.

O- Others such as Listeria monocytogens, B- streptococcus, syphilis.

R- Rubella.

C- Cytomegalovirus.

H- HIV.

CORD BLOOD SAMPLING

Other Names

Cordocentesis, fetal blood sampling, umbilical cord blood testing, and percutaneous umbilical blood sampling (PUBS).

The sampling is done immediately after the delivery.

Even before the delivery the cord blood sampling can be done but the procedure has its own risks and complications involved in such a sampling.

Metabolic disorders are also identified with the help of cord blood sampling. The procedure used for sampling is also used for transfusion of blood to the fetus if there is a necessity for it.

The amount of blood in the Umbilical cord is up to 180mL from a newborn baby that is returned to the neonatal circulation if the umbilical cord is not prematurely clamped. Guided by ultrasound, a thin needle is inserted through the abdominal wall and into the uterus to withdraw a sample of blood from the umbilical cord.

The baby's heartbeat is monitored during the procedure and after the test, breathing and pulse of the mother and the baby's heartbeat are monitored for about an hour and discharged.

Advantages:

Cord blood sampling helps in assessing the acid-base of the fetus.

To rapidly verify the presence of Down syndrome or another fetal chromosomal abnormality.

To evaluate the presence of chromosomal abnormalities when Chorionic Villus Sampling results are ambiguous.

.It allows rapid evaluation of fetal chromosomes when quick decisions must be made about ending the pregnancy or delivering by cesarean section.

To perform a blood count and check for anemia or low platelet levels in the fetus.

Recent studies have shown that cord blood has advantages over traditional bone marrow transplantation, and can be life saving.

The cord blood can be used for the siblings because about 75% of the compatibility has been observed amongst the siblings.

A cord blood bank, used to store umbilical cord blood for future use.

Cord blood contains haematopoietic stem cells, progenitor cells which can form red blood cells, white blood cells and platelets.

Cord blood cells are currently used to treat blood and immune system related genetic diseases, cancers and blood disorders. Medical critics of routine cord blood collection emphasize that neonatal cord blood is physiologically valuable.

Collection of Cord Blood

It is done after the umbilical cord has been cut and the blood is extracted from the placental end of the cord. About 100 to 180 ml of blood is collected, and sent to the laboratory for the analysis. Stem cells from the placenta also can be collected , subjected to testing for viral infections like toxoplasmosis, rubella, or cytomegalovirus in the fetus, HIV, Hepatitis B & C and tissue typing to determine HLA type, cryopreserved for future use at minus 90 degrees Celsius and later frozen at minus 196 degrees Celsius

The collection of cord blood can also be done before the delivery and the procedure is same as that of chorionic villus sampling.

Benefits of Banking Cord Blood

Cord blood stem cells are currently used in the treatment of several life-threatening diseases, and play an important role in the treatment of blood and immune system related genetic diseases, cancers and blood disorders.

The first clinically documented use of cord blood stem cells was in the successful treatment of a six-year-old boy afflicted by Fanconi anemia in 1988. Since then, cord blood has become increasingly recognized as a source of stem cells that can be used in stem cell therapy.

Disadvantages:

The use of autologous cord blood cells for the treatment of childhood leukemia is contra-indicated because pre-leukemic cells are present at birth. Autologous cord blood carries the same genetic defects as the donor and should not be used to treat genetic diseases.

Some of the infections are also identified with such blood samplings Taking samples is done with the help of thin needles that are inserted in the abdomen of the mother and ultrasound is used to guide the procedure for taking the samples.

The fetal vein is used to get the blood sample from the umbilical cord.

Infections after taking the sample and miscarriage are some of the risks associated with sampling.

The presence of maternal blood or amniotic fluid in the sample distorts results.

Pre Implantation

During the morula stage, 1-2 cells are removed from the cleavage stage of the embryo from 'in vitro fertilization' (IVF).

This enables a couple to decide, whether pregnancy should be attempted, rather than terminated at a later stage.

Preimplantation diagnosis is done at various stages in the development of embryo.

a. **POLAR BODY BIOPSY:** After the completion of 1st meiotic division of the oocyte, the nucleus of the 1st polar body, which is a mirror image of the nucleus of secondary oocyte, is examined as it is inactive and does not contribute to the development of embryo.

b. **MULTI CELL BIOPSY:** Before the late 8-cell stage, the blastomere of pre embryo is collected by boring a small hole in the zona pellucida and pipetting the cells. The hole closes and heals quickly. One to three cells are removed by micropipette for analysis.

Blastocyst Biopsy

Human blastocysts containing 60 or more cells programmed for differentiation (totipotent) are used. From trophoblast a number of cells can be safely removed for analysis without adversely affecting the embryo.

Molecular Genetics and Prenatal Diagnosis

Advances in the molecular genetics have made it to diagnose genetic disorders by direct examination of DNA of nucleus – by hybridization and linkage methods- which are used to diagnose genetic disease in any nucleated cell.

New Tissue Aspiration Technique

Transcervical cell collection of foetal cells is done by:

1. Intrauterine lavage
2. Cervical mucus aspiration
3. Cytobrush sampling.

These procedures are done at external OS of cervix uteri.

Intracervical and intrauterine lavage provide foetal nucleated cells but the safty of these techniques have yet to be proven in ongoing pregnencies. The foetal cells, thus obtained by various methods are subjected to

a. *Flow cytometry:* Which is useful only for the determination of the amount of DNA. It will not yield any information about individual chromosomal aneuploidy. It can detect triploidy. Sample required for the flow cytometry is very little , which is 0.1 gm this technique can be applied fixed tissues in paraffin blocks.

b. *Electromicroscopy:* Examples of conditions to be diagnosed with electron microscopy are:

   i. Mitochondrial myopathies
   ii. Viral infections.

24

Chapter

Genetic Counseling

Every year thousands of families are affected by the birth of an abnormal child. About 0.5% of new born have a chromosomal abnormality with moderate to severe phenotypic effects. Another 0.5 – 1.0% suffer the consequences of single gene defects – dominant, recessive or X linked.

About 2% have a malformation that may be due to, in part, heritable factors. Therefore, no doubt about the need for increased genetic information and counseling serves for the many families that require it.

DEFINITION

Genetic counseling is a communication process where individuals seeking advice are provided with scientific information, to enable them to take a decision about current or future pregnancies.

Aim

To convey medical and genetic facts to an affected or potentially affected family in a way that can be understood.

Counseling requires professionals who are thoroughly grounded in both genetics and medicine.

To this basic education, must be added, patience, sensitivity, respect and ability to talk easily with people who are likely to be deeply troubled.

Illness and disability bring tremendous stress to the family life and marriages break if the parents or the children are suffering from genetic defects.

Counselors must be prepared to deal with people who are experiencing denial, shock, anger, despair and guilt.

All this may require the joint efforts of a team of counselors.

The team includes:

1. A clinician with genetic training.
2. A geneticist with mathematical background.
3. Laboratory personnel.
4. Public health nurse.
5. Social worker/genetic associate skilled in working with families in their home environment.

The first **heredity clinic** employing a team approach to genetic counseling was established at the **University of Michigan in 1940**.

Procedure

I. Who needs it?

The need arises when:

1. A child is born with hereditary disorder and the parents and other family members are concerned with the well-being of the future children.
2. Couples may be troubled by repeated abortions or miscarriages.
3. Couples may have heard about greater risk of certain birth defects with advanced maternal age.
4. People without any history of genetic disorder may also want to know whether they are harboring any potentially harmful gene. (This is when there is consanguineous marriage).

II. Medical diagnosis

Genetic counseling requires precise diagnosis because a number of conditions have multiple causes.

In addition to examining the prepositus (Proband), the counselors may want to see other members of the family, or possibly even the family photographs. The clerical work involved in corresponding with relatives and searching for pertinent medical records and autopsy reports is time consuming.

Laboratory work includes, karyotyping, biochemical analysis of blood, urine, cultured cells, molecular analysis etc.

ANY WRONG DIAGNOSIS MAY LEAD TO DEVASTATING CONSEQUENCES!!!

III. Pedigree analysis

There must be 3 to 4 generations of the family obtained. The reliability of the information collected must be assessed. Miscarriages, stillbirths, or mildly affected relatives must be recorded or noted.

IV. Estimating recurrence risks

With the advent of molecular techniques, more and more disease causing Mendelian genes can be analyzed prenatally using fetal cells, obtained through amniocentesis or chorionic villus sampling.

For certain traits, the geographical or racial background of a couple may be an important element of risk estimation.

For many congenital malformations, such as spina bifida, cleft lip or club foot, the risk of recurrence of a particular malformation after the birth of one affected child to normal parents is about 2–5%.

The risk figures must be conveyed in such a way that they can be understood.

V. Options

When genetic prognosis is unfavorable, a couple may refrain from childbearing or risk a defective birth.

If abortion/MTP is an acceptable alternative, it should be advised.

Couple may choose adoption or an appropriate reproductive technology like, artificial insemination or donor egg (ovum).

The perception of risk and willingness of an individual, to accept it are highly subjective matters, depending on one's personality, experiences, moral convictions and especially on the burden of care imposed by the condition. Couple may decide to take a chance on a relatively mild disorder, or on a more serious disorder of a short duration or on one that can be ameliorated by treatment. But they may not be willing to accept the same percentage of risk on a disorder that imposes greater physical, financial and emotional burdens on themselves and their family.

The humanistic aspects of counseling are extremely important because a couple may need time to talk it out between themselves and their relatives and friends. The process should not be hurried.

VI. Follow up and Supportive services

a. A counselor's spoken words may be misinterpreted or forgotten; the relevant medical and genetic information is often put in writing. This includes – names, addresses of specialists and appropriate social services as well as written answers to the major questions raised by the clients.

b. Families should be informed about useful new research results.

c. Relatives, who are unknowingly at risk, may be given proper services.

Overall the entire counselor must provide expert and caring assistance to persons whose self esteem has been hurt and whose life is suddenly complicated by the birth of a child with genetic disorder.

ETHICAL CONCERNS

Generally counselors tell only the truth, all of it, virtually all of it!

The conflict between letting or withholding information is acute with regard to relatives who have not sought counseling. It is still a controversial subject whether to withhold the information and warn the persons of some other consequences to alert them or not. The most important thing is to keep the disease/ disorder confidential and parents and persons actually involved must be informed.

PITFALLS IN GENETIC COUNSELING

1. Incomplete or incorrect diagnosis.
2. Genetic heterogenesity.
3. Non penetrance of the disease.
4. Variable expression of genetic disorder.
5. Inadequate knowledge of literature.
6. Previously undescribed disease.
7. Gonadal mosaicism (genetically distinct cell lines originating from single zygote).

Detailed clinical examination is very essential and a record of all dysmorphic features should be made.

The following are the essential examinations to be conducted:

C = Chromosomal analysis.

A = Autopsy (in case of examination after death).

R = Radiological survey.

P = Photograph of the individual, preferably front and side views of that individual.

25 Chapter GENE THERAPY

It is the correction of effects of abnormal alleles by supplying the normal alleles.

In this, transfer of foreign DNA into the cells is done for therapeutic purposes.

Broken genes in genetic disorders are cut and fixed by a virus. Therefore, "Gene therapy is a technology of introducing foreign genetic material into a patient for correcting genomic defect".

The hope is that the transferred genes will cure the basic defects rather than merely alleviate its damage.

It is rather 'a cure' and the treatment is stopped once the health is regained.

Initially the gene therapy will be used for rectifying a pathogenic condition at a specific site, rather than curing defect in the body ubiquitously.

The best form of delivery or administration would be tissue or cell specific gene transfer.

The gene delivery/administration systems are:

a. Viral.

b. Nonviral.

VIRAL METHODS

Include retrovirus, adenovirus, adeno-associated virus, herpes virus, and vaccinia virus mediated transfer. These are called VECTORS.

NON VIRAL METHODS

Include direct micro injection, electrophoration calcium phosphate, liposome and plasmid based gene transfer.

PROTOCOL

Controlled and elevated levels of transcription in vivo are a fundamental requirement of any gene transfer protocol.

Transfer of novel genes into cells must not harm the cell by the extension of an organism.

TYPES OF GENE THERAPY

There are two types:

1. Somatic gene therapy.
2. Germinal gene therapy.

1. **Somatic gene therapy:** In this, the body cells of the patient receive the corrected gene.
2. **Germinal gene therapy:** In this method of treatment the germ cells of the patient receive the corrected gene.

If the germ cells were also changed from *mutant* to *normal*, the cure could extend through future generations. However, *objections* have been raised to this 'germinal gene therapy' because there will be the possibilities of unwarranted or unwise tampering with another generations of genes.

Therefore, investigations of human gene therapy have been limited to the correction of the disease within individuals and not for the future generations.

This is the traditional aim of medicine. Therefore somatic gene therapy is considered as an ethical option, as long as proper safeguards are in place.

Thus, the proposals for human gene therapy have to pass through many levels of review by government oversight committee. These committees examine ethical issues, safety procedures for the patient and the general public, possible benefit to the patient in relation to the possible risk, because the negative applications of gene therapy are so frightening, that legislation will have to be strictly implemented before making this technology public.

The first federally approved trial on gene therapy to treat a genetic disease was begun in September 1990, at National Institute of Health (NIH). It involved a four-year-old girl with a fatal immunological disease – ADA deficiency.

Till the end of 1995, 106 clinical trials of gene therapy were approved in U.S.

92 of 106 trials have used crippled viruses to carry the genes into the cells.

In many, it caused trouble– some provoked inflammation and destroyed immune system of both virus and virus carrying cell.

Procedure usually involves introduction of pertaining normal DNA into retrovirus; the retrovirus infect the target cells with high efficiency (100%). Then, in the normal course of their virus life cycle, they cause a copy of DNA of their genetic material to be inserted into the chromosomal DNA of the host cell.

One retrovirus available for human gene therapy is the mouse leukemia virus. Before using it, the researchers remove most of the genetic material of the virus to render it incapable of further reproduction. The empty space in the viral RNA is then replaced with suitable human RNA. This substitution does not affect the ability of the virus to:

i. Infect human cells.

ii Insert a DNA copy of its genetic material into the cells' DNA.

The other organisms used as VECTORS are:

1. E. coli.
2. Cosmids or plasmids.
3. Baker's yeast.
4. Bacteriophage or phage cells.

HURDLES IN THE TECHNOLOGY OF GENE THERAPY

1. Gene corrected T-cell therapy depends on a basic concept of immune system in some genetic diseases. A single T-cell or B-cell is programmed to respond to just one antigen and such competent immune cells, which are needed to mount an attack against some antigens of disease causing microbes, may be missing.

To overcome this problem, the stem cells of the bone marrow are obtained and one time injection of these cells is enough to cure the disease.

2. The insertion of the retrovirus borne gene into T-cell appears to be at random places in the genome rather than at the locus of the abnormal gene. There is a risk of interruption of some normal gene activities or death of the cells.
3. The infectious viruses may be generated and spread to other cells.

PROTOCOLS FOR GENE THERAPY

Usually they are done in experimental animals. Plenty of experiments are being conducted and the results are awaited.

1. Use of retroviruses on extracted cells.
2. Introduction of gene carrying virus directly to the body.
3. Injection of DNA itself.

Since the knowledge of inner workings of the cells is still fragmentary and many biological examples could be of well intentioned, interventions produce unexpected side effects.

SOME 'GENE THERAPY' PROPOSALS IN EARLY CLINICAL TRIALS/NEAR APPROVED STAGES

DISEASE		*DESCRIPTION OF THERAPY.*
1. ADA- deficiency	:	T-cells extracted from patient, gene Corrected and returned by retrovirus vector or same as above but using bone marrow stem cells.
2. Familial hyperchole- -sterolemia	:	Liver cells from patient corrected sterolemia for LDL receptor gene by retroviral vector and reintrodu- ced.
3. Cystic fibrosis	:	Adenovirus (cold virus) carrying Normal CFTR gene introduced Directly into airways of patient by an aerosol spray.
4. Duchene muscular	:	Direct injection of dystrophin gene dystrophy into muscle cells.

5. Cardiovascular disease : Cells lining blood vessels altered to stick to the arterial walls and produce clot dissolving protein.
6. Skin cancer : Melanomas injected with a gene in a plasmid that produces a protein to stimulate the immune system to attack the cancer. No cells are removed from the body.
7. Gene therapy is given to cure baldness, wrinkles of the skin of the face and body and also aging.
8. DEGF2 gene is used to cure vascular disorders. Genes are used to regenerate tissues.
9. Injected vascular endothelial factor at the site of vascular damage in necrosed/infracted heart wall lead to formation of new vessels after 8 weeks and in 6 months there was complete vascularisation.
10. Adenovirus is a large double helical DNA virus which is engineered to destroy NS tumors (Non spreading).

RETROVIRUSES ENCLOSE AN RNA MOLECULE AND HAVE BEEN TESTED FOR SUPPRESSING VARIETY OF MALIGNANT NEOPLASMS

The viral methods:

1. Require cell receptors for the entry of virus particles.
2. Successful retroviral induction depends on ability to induce proliferation in cells at least for a short time.
3. The purification of viral particles may lead to significant loss of infectivity.
4. Ability of the cells to perpetuate an infection and spread virus to the other cells.
5. Non contamination of cellular RNAs packaged into retroviral vectors.

To conclude, gene therapy may finally become useful adjunct to treat life threatening diseases but may not wholly replace the currently practised protocols, but, gene has the same side effect as any other drug has the side effect, therefore, gene therapy has its own limitations.

26 Chapter DERMATOGLYPHICS

It is a Greek word, in which 'Derma' is 'Skin' and 'Glyph' means 'Carving'.

This is a science which deals with the study of dermal ridge configuration on the digits, palms, toes and soles.

These patterns start developing as early as 13th week of intrauterine life and complete by 19th week of intrauterine life. Once formed, they do not change till death.

Walker was the first person to demonstrate the typical pattern in case of Down syndrome.

Even if a specific syndrome may not be diagnosed, still it seems to be a useful screening procedure, specifically in Down syndrome. Abnormal pattern has some diagnostic value as a sign of disturbed prenatal growth, e.g., in cases of mental retardation whether the cause is perinatal or prenatal.

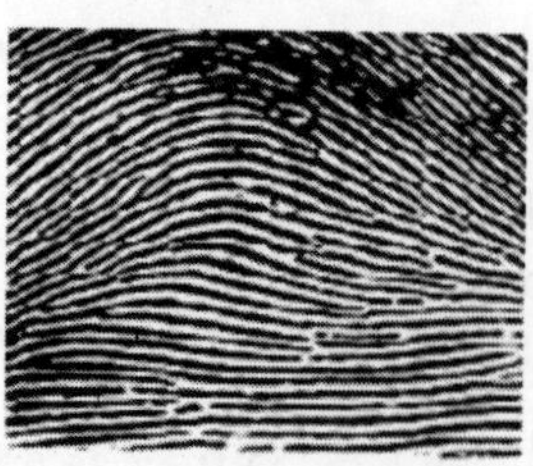

Arch

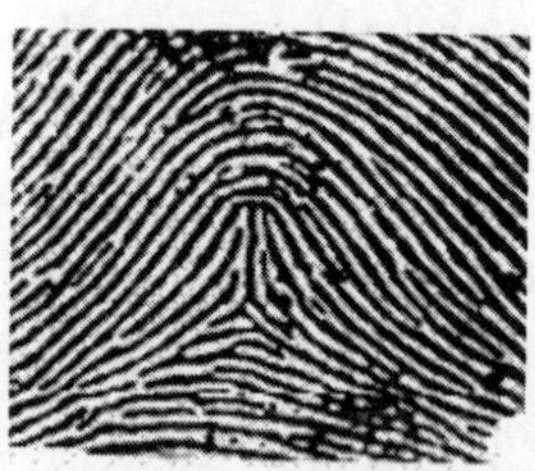

Tented arch

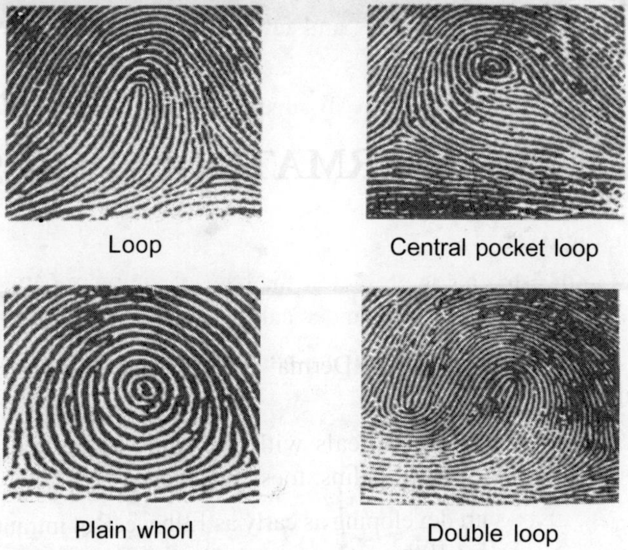

Fig. 26.1: Various finger tip ridge patterns

Each fingerprint is composed of between 50 and 100 lines. Though no two fingerprints are exactly alike, prints can be classified into one of 4 major types: the whorl, the loop, the arch and the tented arch.

TERMINOLOGIES USED

I. Finger tip pattern: They are of 3 to 4 types, classified by the number of 'triradii' present. Triradius is a point present at the confluence of ridges going in different directions like a fork.

1. **Simple arch:** Has no triradius.
2. **Tented arch:** Has central triradius.
3. **Loop:** Has single triradius and is called 'ULNAR' or 'RADIAL', depending on the side to which it opens.
4. **Whorl:** Has two or more triradii: may be double loop or more commonly a circular type of pattern.

Total Ridge Count (TRC): It is done from centre of the pattern up to the farthest triradius.

- Arches have ZERO TRC.

- Whorls have HIGHEST TRC.

Females have more arches and few whorls than in males. There are racial differences also.

II. Palmar pattern: They are divided into:

1. Thenar area.
2. Hypothenar area.
3. Interdigital area.

Normally triradius is present at the base of the palm between the thenar and hypothenar areas and is called AXIAL TRIRADIUS.

The four interdigital triradii are named –'a, b, c and d'.

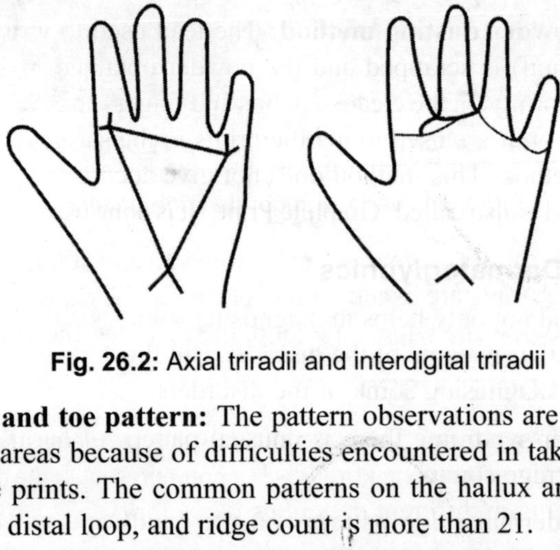

Fig. 26.2: Axial triradii and interdigital triradii

III. Sole and toe pattern: The pattern observations are confined to hallucial areas because of difficulties encountered in taking the foot prints/toe prints. The common patterns on the hallux are the whorl and large distal loop, and ridge count is more than 21.

The arch tibial is typically seen in Down syndrome.

IV. Flexion creases: These are dermal attachments to the underlying structures. Appear between 7th and 14th week of intrauterine life.

In the palm there are distal and proximal transverse creases and one thenar crease.

In case of Down syndrome, there is only one crease on the palm and is called SIMIAN crease. The sole will have ARCH TIBIAL patterns in Down syndrome. There is another crease which is single and is proximal transverse crease. It is called SYDNEY LINE.

METHODS OF OBTAINING DERMATOGLYPHIC PATTERN

1. Use of magnifying glass—Temporary.
2. Ink-Pad method—Kores duplicating ink is used because it dries quickly.
3. Lead powder dusting method: Graphite print.
4. Plastic sheet method.

Ink-Pad method: Person is asked to wash hands, with soap and water thoroughly to remove dust, dirt and oil. Stamp pad ink or Kores duplicating ink (4746- Black) is smeared on both hands and prints are taken by rolling the hands from wrist crease to the finger tip, on the roller covered with bond paper.

Lead powder dusting method: The lead used to write (graphite or lead pencil) is scrapped and the powder obtained, is smeared or dusted uniformly on the cleaned palms and fingers and the roller along with paper on it are used to get the prints in the same way as that of ink-pad method. This method does not give accuracy, so not in use. This method is also called 'Graphite Print'. It is done usually in children.

Uses of Dermatoglyphics

This method not only helps in diagnosing some genetic diseases, but also is peculiar in some of the diseases. But this alone does not form a basis for diagnosing some of the disorders.

In Turner syndrome there is unusual pattern of dermatoglyphics with high ridge count.

The epidermal ridge patterns on the hands and soles are fully developed at birth and thereafter remain unchanged for life. Scanning of the ridge patterns or recording their permanent impressions, i.e., prints can be accomplished rapidly, inexpensively and without any trauma to the patient.

SIMIAN CREASE

The proximal and distal transverse creases are replaced by or joined into one single crease that traverses the whole palm. This single transverse flexion crease is referred to as SIMIAN crease.

The term is inappropriate as it does not represent characteristic palmar crease configuration among apes and monkeys. Only pavian monkey shows this crease.

This crease is also termed as 'single upper palmar crease/single transverse fold / four finger line'.

Simian crease has medical diagnostic value. Popich and Smith (1970) attempted to account for the embryonic development of a single transverse crease on the basis of location and nature of the early fetal interdigital pads. According to their hypothesis, the transverse palmar crease is influenced by both the sloping alignment of the third to fifth metacarpal-phalangeal joints and the nature of the fetal interdigital pads at the time of crease development.

There are variants of this single transverse crease– short, long, split line etc.

This crease is usually associated with the chromosomal anomaly, Trisomy 21 (Down syndrome).

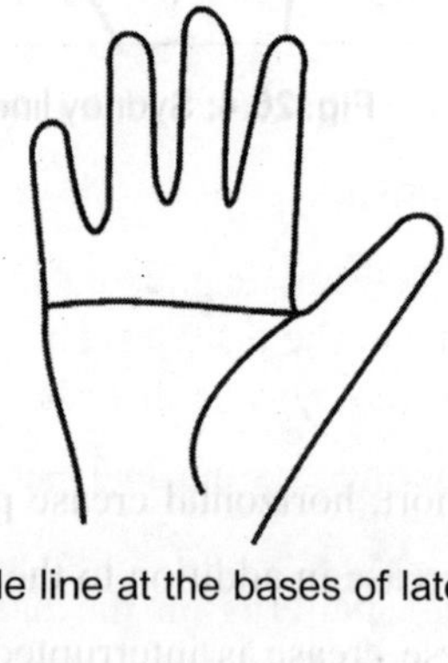

Fig. 26.3: Single line at the bases of lateral four digits

SYDNEY LINE

It is named after the city in Australia where it was observed by PURVIS-SMITH AND MENSER in 1968.

Definition: The proximal palmar crease extends towards the ulnar margin of the palm past the midline axis of the fifth finger.

This line represents a proximal transverse crease that extends beyond the hypothenar eminence to the ulnar margin of the palm. The distal transverse crease persists and appears normal. This extended proximal crease was described earlier by ERNE (1953) and corresponds to special form 1 of WENINGER and NAVRATIL (1957).

In LEIBER's classification (1960) of main palmar creases, the Sydney line is not considered to be a significant abnormality. Later, an increased frequency of the Sydney line was reported in individuals with Down syndrome, congenital rubella and leukemia.

This line was most frequently seen in series of children with delayed development, learning difficulties or minor behavioral problems.

Distal to the Sydney line there is distal palmar crease present on the palm, separate from the lengthened proximal crease.

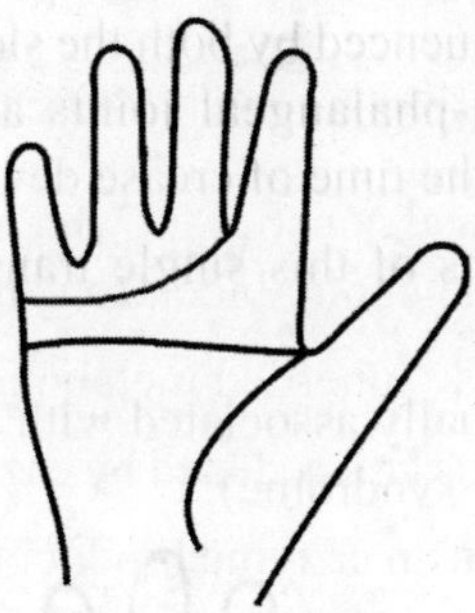

Fig. 26.4: Sydney line

Variations

A. Arching.

B. Double branch.

C. Wide arching.

D. Interrupted and short, horizontal crease present above the gap.

E. Third horizontal crease in addition to the distal crease.

F. Proximal transverse crease is interrupted, cascading to the ulnar border of the palm.

27 Chapter
INBORN ERRORS OF METABOLISM

It is part of biochemical genetics, in which there is a specific enzyme defect, produces a metabolic block to cause pathological effects.

This is also termed "Inherited metabolic disease".

All metabolic events are mediated by enzymes under genetic control.

Thus, a mutation in an enzyme producing gene is likely to induce a metabolic block in one step of a biochemical pathway.

The consequences of an excess of precursors or lack of end products lead to the errors in metabolism.

An English physician and biochemist, Archibald Garrod, first proposed the occurrence of gene-determined inborn errors of metabolism and described several examples of cases in humans, in the beginning of 20th century.

The enzymic disorders are inherited as RECESSIVE TRAITS.

Since 1950, the discovery of metabolic diseases has increased greatly. At least 250 different human metabolic disorders are known.

This is probably because there are newer methods for identifying metabolites and enriched by molecular techniques.

Pharmacogenetics and ecogenetics deal with inherited enzyme variants that lead to individual differences in the metabolism of drugs, diet or other environmental substances.

DETECTION OF METABOLIC DISORDERS IN NEWBORNS

Certain symptoms tend to be common to a wide variety of metabolic disorders. Because some syndromes can be treated, if recognized early, it is very important to be alert to these diagnostic signals. Many affected babies appear normal at birth but very soon develop severe problems.

SOME MOST TELLING SIGNS OF METABOLIC DISORDERS

1. Severe vomiting, beginning in the first few days of life.
2. An abnormal odor to the urine, skin or breath.
3. Abnormal concentrations of ketones or acids in body fluids.
4. Abnormalities in pigment development.
5. Seizures, especially when accompanied by muscle spasms in particular areas of the body.
6. Failure of muscle coordination.

PHYSICAL SIGNS AND POSSIBLE SIGNIFICANCE

Physical Signs		*Possible Significance*
1. Hepatosplenomegaly	:	Amino acid, Organic acid disorders, Lysosomal storage disease
2. Coarse facies	:	Mucopolysaccharidosis e.g. Hurler's syndrome, Gangliosidoses, Mannosidoses
3. Mental retardation	:	Homocysteinuria, Phenylketonuria, Tryptophanuria
4. Failure to thrive	:	Aminoaciduria, organic aciduria, Cysteinuria, Lactic acidosis, Storage diseases
5. Low WBC and low platelets	:	Organic acidurias

Therefore, inborn errors of metabolism will have:

- Common acute presentation
- Diarrhea
- Lethargy
- Respiratory distress
- Metabolic acidosis

- Jaundice
- Hypoglycemia
- Urea and electrolyte imbalance
- Fits
- Coma.

SOME OF THE DISORDERS ASSOCIATED WITH VARIOUS METABOLISMS

I. Amino acid metabolism:

A. Maple sugar urine disease

B. Ornithine transcarbamylase deficiency

C. Phenylketonuria

D. Leucinosis

E. Alkaptonuria

F. Albinism

G. Homocysteinuria

II. Carbohydrate metabolism:

A. Hereditary fructose intolerance

B. Galactosemia

C. Glycogen storage disease

D. Pentosuria

III. Nucleic acid metabolism:

A. ADA deficiency

B. Gout

IV. Organic acid metabolism:

A. Glutaric academia type I

B. MCAD deficiency

V. Lipoprotein and lipid metabolism:

A. Gaucher's disease

B. Familial LCAT deficiency

C. Tay Sach's disease

D. Neiman Pick's disease

E. Essential hypercholesterolemia

VI. Metal metabolism:

A. Hemochromatosis (Iron metabolism)

B. Menkes (steely hair) disease

C. Wilson's disease (Copper metabolism)

VII. Lysosomal enzymes:

A. Mucopolysaccharidosis I

B. Mucopolysaccharidosis II

C. Gaucher disease type I

VIII. Peroxisomal enzymes:

A. Adrenoleukodystrophy

B. Zellweger syndrome.

IX. Hormone metabolism:

A. X linked icthyosis

B. Goitrous cretinism

X. Blood protein metabolism:

A. Von Willebrand disease I

B. Hemophilia

XI. Connective tissue protein metabolism:

A. Osteogenesis imperfecta type I

B. Ehlers Danlos syndrome type IV

C. Marfan syndrome

XII. Defects in purine and pyrimidine metabolism.

A. Gout

B. Juvenile hyperuricemia

C. Xanthuria

XIII. Defects in membrane transport:

A. Renal glycosuria

B. Glucose-Galactose malabsorption

C. Cysteinuria

D. Hartnup disease

E. Phosphaturia

XIV. Defects in lysosomal enzyme

Accumulation of mucopolysaccharides in connective tissue–Hurler's syndrome, Hunter's syndrome and Fucosidosis.

28 Chapter

HUMAN GENOME PROJECT

Genome is the entire collection of chromosomes present in the nucleus of each cell of all individual organisms. Human genome has 24 different chromosomes (22 allosomes and X & Y sex chromosomes). They contain 3 billion nucleotides and range in size from 45 million to 279 million Pb (pair base).

Genomics is a branch of biology which deals with the study of whole genomes, is dedicated to the development and application of more effective mapping, sequencing and computational tools.

Genomics use large scale or global molecular techniques for linkage analysis, physical mapping and sequencing of genomes, to generate vast amount of data, which can be analyzed by computer.

Sophisticated programmes enable geneticists to predict existence and in some cases, general functions of previous undefined genes.

Molecular biologists can then confirm the computer generated projections through biochemical studies and genetic engineering in model organisms. The model organisms used in genomic analysis have many genetic mechanisms and cellular pathways in common with each other and with humans.

In 1985, a meeting on the project took place in Santa Cruz, California. Twelve biologists of diverse background were assembled to explore the idea of starting an institute to sequence the human genome. After two days deliberations, they concluded that it is possible to develop the technology required to accomplish this.

Two important ideas were put forward:

1. Concepts of human genome project introduced the idea of discovery

of science– a new scientific approach to biology in discovery science one seeks to identify all elements of biological system, e.g., Complete sequence of 24 chromosomes that has 3 million nucleotides in human genome and place them in a data base to enrich the infrastructure of biology and can be used for biological analysis. The science stands in contrast to hypothesis driven approach to biology.

2. Human genomic project required the development of high through put. Automated DNA sequence technology, as well as computational tools is necessary for capturing, storing and analyzing vast amount of cloning, mapping and sequence data associated with obtaining genome sequences. This needs integrating the ENGINEERING, COMPUTER SCIENCE, PHYSICS, MATHEMATICS and BIOLOGY, leading to cross disciplinary approach that would eventually transform modern biology and genetics. Earlier, it was thought that only 2% of the genome represented genes and 98% was junk.

In 1988, National Academy of Science appointed committee– half proponents and half opponents– to consider the scientific merits of human genome project (HGP). After one year the committee unanimously endorsed the project.

The United States government funded HGP in 1990 with a projected 15-year scale and three million dollar budget for completing human genome sequence. The HGP was launched to read the 3 billion nucleotide long human DNA base by base. The goals of this mega science project are:

1. Creation of genetic maps.
2. Development of physical maps.
3. Determination of complete human DNA sequence.

To facilitate the analysis of human genome, small sets of model organisms like bacterium, yeast, nematode, worm, fruit fly and laboratory mouse have also been put up for sequencing assignment.

Objects of Human Genome Project: There are six distinct objects. They are:

1. To generate physical, genetic and sequence maps of human genome.

2. To sequence genomes of a variety of model organisms.
3. To develop improved technology for mapping and sequencing.
4. To develop computational tools for capturing, storing, analyzing, displaying, and distributing map and sequence information.
5. To sequence EST fragments of cDNAs (EST= Expressed Sequence Tags are single sequence runs– 600 pb on the cDNA inserts) and eventually full length cDNAs encoding the expressed mRNAs in different cell types of human and mice. (cDNA= copy or complimentary DNA).
6. To consider the ethical, social and legal challenges posed by genomic information.

A rough sequence draft of the human genome was completed in February 2001.The final sequence was completed in 2003. Eight model organisms identified– E. coli.

This helped to identify more than 1000 genes causing different human diseases.

This identification helps for diagnosis and treatment. More than 4 million human and 2 million mice EST have been sequenced.

EST and cDNA sequences are playing an important role in defining gene locations, alternate RNA splicing patterns, exon/intron boundaries in Genomic sequences.

cDNA: Because most of the DNA (about 97%) does not code for proteins, tRNA or rRNA; cDNA is transcribed from mRNA and contains essentially the coding triplets for the amino acids of cell proteins. In cDNA there are no introns.

POST GENOMIC ERA

Biologists may, one day understand the molecular basis of every genetic disease, as well as networks of molecular interactions that brings every person to life in a unique way.

Social and personal repercussions of the information gained from genomic analysis are generating new areas of biological concerns. The HGP seeks to sequence all 3 billion bases of our DNA in a coordinated international effort. To avoid sequencing long tracts of repetitive or intronic DNA (97%), some investigators may make use of cDNA.

The mapping and sequencing of human genome will provide extensive new knowledge about the genes involved in inherited diseases, birth defects, late onset diseases with a genetic component including heart diseases, neurological disorders and behavioral disorders, many forms of cancer and even susceptibility to infection. This knowledge will have profound impact on the understanding, detection, prevention and treatment of these disorders.

Interest in the Human Genome Project is centered in Europe, Japan and United States under the umbrella of the Human Genome Mapping Organization (HUGO).

In the U.S. organizational and financial support comes from the National Institute of Health and the Department of Energy. James Watson was the first to head the National Center for Human Genome Research.

The approximate number of bases in three different genomes and in some cloning vectors, compared to the number of characters in Webster's unabridged dictionary. (There is a mention of 26000 characters per page – 2770 pages – for a total of 72 million characters!!).

Average insert cloned in a plasmid, phage or cosmid = 30,000 bases= 1 page.

Large insert cloned in a YAC = 1,000,000 bases= 40 pages.

E.coli genome = 5,000,000 bases= 200 pages.

Fruit fly genome= 160,000,000 bases=2 dictionaries = 5,600 pages.

Human genome= 3,000,000,000 bases = 42 dictionaries = 116,000 pages.

Identifying, isolating and analyzing genes is of paramount importance to NIP THE DISEASE IN ITS GENETIC BUD!!

Mapping: This means assigning a particular gene its chromosomal address, i.e., what exact position does it occupy in a chromosome.

A single recognizable chromosome band represents a DNA length of approximately 10 million base pairs. Thus, the progressive narrowing down of this region is the surest way to reach the locus.

The most recently published map of human genome shows 5264 micro satellite markers each separated by a distance of 0.7 cm.

An important GOAL of HGP is to construct a physical map of such 30,000 evenly distributed landmarks distanced at an average space of 100 kilo bases (1 kilo base = 1000 bases).

Physical mapping is done by various techniques which are as follows:

a. Meiotic.

b. Radiation hybrid (RH).

c. In Situ Hybridization (ISH).

d. Sequence tagged sites (STS) contents.

e. Clone based fingerprint mapping (FM).

DNA SEQUENCING

The most challenging task for HGP researchers is to develop a technology for RAPID, ACCURATE and COST EFFECTIVE DNA sequencing of large genomes.

Automation has enabled faster DNA sequencing at reduced cost and with greater accuracy.

It has been found that many genes in the lower organisms appreciably resemble DNA sequences of higher eukaryocytes.

HGP was proposed in 1990 with a projected 15 years scale (upto 2005), but it was completed by 2003.

PROTEOMICS

Protein coding genes generate proteomics. From draft sequence of human genome, investigators predicted more than 30,000 protein coding genes. The collective translation of the 30,000 predicted genes into proteins are termed the proteomes.

Human proteome contain homologs– In the context, protein related by evolutionary descent – for 61% of the fruit fly proteome. Proteomic analysis have revealed that there are about 1200 gene families containing two or more members, 92 (7%) of which are vertebrate specific. These vertebrate specific families encode proteins active in immunity, other types of defence, and the nervous system. Analysts have also shown that there has been a striking increase in complexity of the proteome from yeast to animals, this increase in complexity has come about in five ways.

1. More genes – Human has more genes than model organism.
2. The shuffling increase or decrease of functional modules – Human organism has only modest increase in the total no. of protein domains over the model organisms, it has evolved many new gene arrangements that alter domain architecture.
3. More paralogs – Human has 1000 olfactory genes whereas fish has only 60.
4. Alternate RNA splicing.
5. Chemical modification of proteins.

Human cell might have 20,000 different type of mRNA and perhaps 200000 different proteins.

By all these criteria human proteomics is considerably more complex than its counterparts in the fly, worm or yeast.

Evolution may occur by the lateral transfer of genes from one organism to another. Lateral gene transfer is the direct transfer of genes from species into germ line of another species. About 200 such human genes are there.

The possibility of lateral gene transfer suggests that, in principle, evolutionary potential of one species is enormously enhanced by access to successful evolutionary strategies of other species- It also adds fuel to the debate over genetic engineering, providing a counterpoint to the argument that humans are genetically unique. Different human races appear to have very few unique distinguishing genes. For example Phenotypic features like skin color, skin fold at the corners of eye.

The sequences of the human and model organism genome reaffirms that all living organisms evolved from a common ancestor.

In future, other features of chromosomes will become increasingly important, Like:

- Chemical modification of bases.
- Interaction of various proteins with chromosomes.
- Three-dimensional nucleus in chromosome.

Conclusion

"High throughput **Genomic** and proteomic platforms permit the global analysis of gene products."

HGP has given us the complete sequences of a variety of genomes. The next step is to carry out global analysis of this basic data to gain a more complete understanding of how cells and larger biological systems use genetic information to create a whole organism.

A high throughput **genomic** platform might include:

1. Automated instrumentation to prepare DNA fragments for sequencing.
2. An automated sequencer to carry out the sequencing, and
3. A set of computational tools to capture and store information obtained from sequencing.

Genomics – to mean global analysis of chromosomal and RNA features such as sequence, genetic marker, mRNA.

Proteomics – to mean global analysis of complex protein mixtures.

Finally the preceding view of medicine in 21st century raises a host of pressing questions about privacy of genetic information, limitations on the use of genetic testing, Patenting the DNA sequences, Society's view of older people, training the physicians and the extent of which the human genetic engineering should seek to engineer himself or herself.

The physician trained today will be practising predictive/preventive medicine in 20 years.

How should their training change to prepare them for new ways of thinking about medicine?

Social and ethical concerned raised by genetic engineering, the ability to alter specific genes of an organism in specific ways.

- Somatic gene therapy.
- Insertion/replacing faulty gene.
- Germ line gene therapy.
- Modifying human germ line.

Many support somatic gene therapy but oppose germ line gene therapy so, serious and open discussion of the issues before perfection of the technology overtakes our ability to control its use.

29 Chapter CODOMINANT GENES (ALLELES)

When both alleles of a pair of chromosomes are expressed in heterozygote state, the alleles are said to be CODOMINANT. They jointly contribute to a given phenotype without diminishing each others activity.

Example is ABO blood group system. The antibodies anti A and anti B are used to determine the presence or absence of the corresponding antigens on red blood cells and many other cell types in the body. The antigens A, B, AB and O of the ABO gene are controlled by A, B, AB and O of ABO gene. The symbol 'A' can be used to indicate an antigen, an antibody, a blood type (phenotype) or an allele (genotype). The context in which the symbol is used makes clear which is meant. The blood types A,B and O correspond to genotype A/B and O/O respectively. Blood types A and B can result either from the corresponding homozygote or from heterozygous combination with the 'O' allele. Thus O allele is recessive to A and B whereas A and B alleles are codominant to each other. The specific genotype for phenotypes A and B can be inferred from the blood types of related individuals. Anti A antibody is found in serum of persons of blood type B or O; anti B in persons of blood group A or O. The blood groups are defined in terms of antigens on the surface of RBCs.

30

Chapter

Gene Mapping or Linkage Analysis

The genes on the same chromosomes that are fairly close to each other are said to be linked. Although the genes are physically located on the same chromosome, tend to be inherited together, they can recombine with their alleles on the homologous chromosomes by their remarkable process. Genes on the same chromosome are connected to each other like two knots spaced along a rope, or two links on a chain, or two rings on a raccoon's tail. The genes (knots, rings or chains) need not be next to each other. They are still physically bound together through intervening sections.

All the genes on a chromosome are attached in series, like successive kilometer sections on a highway, it is a long and narrow chromosomal highway. In theory, each gene can be mapped with respect to its near neighbors and those neighbors; with respect to additional neighbors to yield the relative position of the perhaps 2000 X linked genes.

Like distances along a highway, the distances along the chromosomes are also additive, for example, a and b = 4 units apart, b and c = 8 units apart and a and c are 12 units apart when a,b,c..... genes are in that order in that chromosome.

The Significance of Gene Mapping

The construction of human gene map can be likened to the assembly of a jigsaw puzzle. Initially there is a disorder. Then border pieces are separated from inside pieces.

Locating a gene is often a prerequisite to isolating and cloning it, which in turn lead to information about the encoded protein. The knowledge of human diseased gene and its protein product brings us the much closer to early diagnosis and treatment.

Gene mapping can also help detect or explain multiple causes of the similar genetic disease, e.g., abnormal blood clotting occurs due to many different reasons related to mutant genes at different X linked and autosomal loci. Proper therapy requires the knowledge of the exact cause of the defect.

Comparative genome mapping is an active and exciting area of research. Most similar human karyotypes are those of chimpanzee, gorilla, and orangutan – all having 48 chromosomes. Comparisons of banding patterns among these four species reveal, virtually identical X chromosomes and remarkable similarity of autosomes as well. Only the Y chromosomes vary considerably from species to species. Comparison of mammalian gene locations and chromosome banding patterns provide information on evolutionary sequences.

For two genes nearby on the same chromosome, a double heterozygote can still make four types of gametes, but their proportions will not be 1/4 each. The proportions of parental and recombinant gametes from such linked genes will depend on:

a. Physical distance separating two genes along the chromosomes.
b. Whether the double heterozygote is in the coupling or repulsion phase.

Microscopically visible chiasmata represent the positions of crossing over events, exact exchanges of pieces of non sister chromatid. Crossing over provides a measure of physical distance along a chromosome. This equivalence is reasonably accurate as long as recombination is under about 25%, in which case X% of recombination is defined as X map units.

Gene mapping can be done in human X chromosome by looking at the phenotype of the sons of doubly heterozygous mothers. The phenotype of each son reflects the genetic constitution of the egg from which he arose.

Chromosomes can be mapped in recombination units or located to specific stained band by family linkage studies or by somatic cell and molecular techniques.

Mapping information provides fundamental knowledge of genome organization and has practical applications in genetic counseling, medicine and agriculture.

31 Chapter

Philadelphia Chromosome

Structural change in a chromosome can contribute to cancer induction. This discovery was first made in 1960 at the University of Pennsylvania in Philadelphia and focused on the role of the socalled Philadelphia chromosome in Leukemia (Chronic Myeloid Leukemia). It affects mainly people of middle age and older age and is invariably fatal. It is easily recognized because the leukemic cells usually have a distinctive chromosomal marker, the Philadelphia chromosome, which is a shortened chromosome 22, originally thought to result from a simple deletion.

The introduction of banding techniques revealed that end pieces of long arms of chromosomes 9 and 22 – unequal in size – had switched places through a reciprocal translocation. The regions around the break point of chromosomes 9 and 22 have been cloned and sequenced. The break point in chromosome 9 occurs in the cellular parts of oncogene – c – abl. The break point in chromosome 22 occurs in a gene called the breakage cluster region (BCR), but the specific function is not known. The fused gene in Philadelphia chromosome is transcribed and translated into an abnormally long protein whose immediate effect in cells is a matter of speculation.

The reciprocal translocation between chromosome 9 and 22 that produces the Philadelphia chromosome, characteristic of chromosome myeloid leukemia. Breakage and reunion join together the L-abl proto-oncogene on chromosome 9 with a socalled breakage cluster region on chromosome 22.

The leukemias occur with increased incidence among radiologists exposed to excessive amounts of X radiation, among patients receiving large doses of therapeutic radiation and among the people exposed to atomic bomb explosion.

THE PHILADELPHIA CHROMOSOME

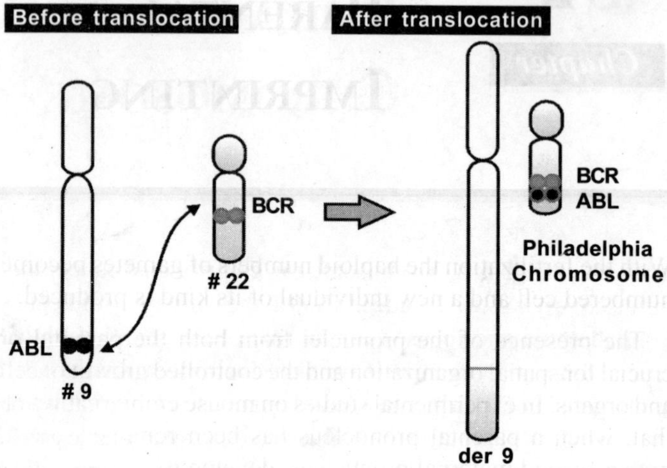

Fig. 31.1: Philadelphia chromosome showing reciprocal translocation

32 Chapter

PARENTAL IMPRINTING

With the fertilization the haploid numbers of gametes become diploid numbered cell and a new individual of its kind is produced.

The presence of the pronuclei from both the parental origins is crucial for spatial organization and the controlled growth of cell, tissues and organs. In experimental studies on mouse embryo, it was observed that, when a parental pronucleus has been removed, and replaced with a second maternal pronucleus, develop to a relatively advanced stage (25 pairs of somites), but with limited development of trophoblast. In contrast embryos in which the maternal pronucleus has been replaced by a second parental pronucleus, develop very poorly forming embryo of only 6 to 8 somites, but with an extensive trophoblast. Thus, it appears that the maternal genome is relatively more important for the development of the embryo whereas the paternal genome is essential for the development of extraembryonic tissues that lead to placental formation.

This functional inequivalence of homologous paternal chromosomes is called 'parental imprinting'. The process of parental imprinting causes the expression of particular genes to be independent on their parental origin, with some genes being expressed only from maternally inherited chromosome and others from paternally inherited chromosome. These genes are called 'imprinted genes'. They are believed to have inherited maternal or paternal specific imprints which affect their activity.

The mechanism of imprinting is thought to involve the acquisition of molecular signals attached to the DNA or chromatin which are known as epigenetic modifications. These modifications must have the following properties:

1. They must be able to affect the transcription of the gene.
2. They must be inheritable in somatic cells over many cell divisions and not lost during chromosome replication.
3. Most importantly the imprints must be erased in the male and be female germ lines during gametogenesis to allow new imprints to be set down which are specific to the parental origin of the newly formed gametes.

Methylation of critical CpG dinucleotides in DNA of imprinted genesis one type of epigenetic modification believed to be important in the imprinting process.

The requirement for both parental genomes is limited to a subset of the chromosomes. This has become evident through the analysis of individuals with uniparental duplications and corresponding deficiencies of particular chromosomal regions, uniparental disomy. The uniparental disomy can arise through meiotic and mitotic nondisjunction events and results in individuals completely disomic or exhibiting mosaicism of disomic and nondisomic cells. If imprinted genes reside on the affected chromosomes then the uniparental disomic cells will either express a double dose of gene or have both copies repressed.

In human some conditions show parental origin effects in their patterns of inheritance and several imprinted disorders in man have been described. These disorders can be attributed to the alterations in the dosage of imprinted genes either through chromosomal uniparental disomy, trisomy or mutations like deletions involving gene or the imprints. In these disorders, both male and female are equally affected. However, a manifestation of the disorder depends on the parental origin of the uniparental disomy or the sex of the parent from whom the mutation is inherited. The disorders which exhibit parental origin effecting in their patterns of inheritance are – Beckwith - Wiedemann syndrome, Prader-willi syndrome and Angelman syndrome.

Parental imprinting mutations are also implicated in the genesis of some tumor syndromes like Wilms tumor and Familial glomus tumors.

33 Chapter HOMEOBOX GENES (HOX GENES)

One of a subgroup of homeobox genes that are found in clusters on the genes of vertebrates. These are referred to as Hox clusters in mammals. Hox clusters play a role in directing embryonic development (Homeo-alike).

Over many decades embryologists have described in detail the changes and interactions of specific embryonic cells during development from single cell (zygote) and orderly course of differentiation. Studies in fruit fly embryos indicate that two kinds of gene families control the development. They are:

a. Maternal effect genes.

b. Segmentation genes and pattern formation genes.

A. MATERNAL EFFECT GENES

Help in everything needed for cleavage division, nucleotides and enzymes for DNA replication, tubulin for spindle formation, constituents needed for protein synthesis, ribosomes, messenger RNA molecules which encode genetic information, transcribed from maternal DNA. These gene products will give rise to head to tail, and front to back axes in developing embryo.

B. SEGMENTATION AND PATTERN FORMATION GENES

These genes become activated by maternal formation gene and takeover from maternal formation genes. First, segmentation genes interact with one another to subdivide the embryo into regions. Then pattern forming genes assign a regional identity to each resulting domain – repeated patterns along the length of the embryo.

Such pattern formation occurs through the action of the socalled, homeotic genes which act by naming or specifying the structures unique to each subunit. Using molecular techniques, geneticists isolated and sequenced the genes and gene products of some segmentation and homeotic loci. All were found to be complex and interrelated. They shared similar sequence of 180DNA base factors which were termed the HOMEOBOX GENES (HOX GENES).

A homeobox in a DNA is a sequence found within genes that are involved in the regulation of development of animals, fungi and plants. Genes that have a homeobox are called homeobox genes. They form the homeobox gene family.

The segmentation takes place in CNS, muscles and back bones. These HOMEOBOX sequences have remained highly conserved throughout evolution. Fruit flies have about 10 HOMEOBOX (HOX) genes on chromosome 3. In humans and mice about 40 HOX genes have been identified, distributed among four different gene complexes on separate chromosomes.

In vertebrates, embryonic and regenerating limbs are good subjects for analyzing the homeobox proteins. Thus, many of the genes known from mutations to be essential for normal embryonic morphology had one small region in common – the homeobox – that code for a DNA binding functions.

By controlling the transcription in all cells, **homeobox (Hox) genes act as master switches determining cell fates, growth, and development**.

Currently thirtyeight genes containing HOMEOBOXES are known in mammals and all show a high degree of similarity with homeoboxes of the Drosophila homeotic genes. These genes are Hox (murine), HOX (human) are found in four clusters known as:

A. Mouse chromosome 6 — Human chromosome 7
B. Mouse chromosome 11 — Human chromosome 17
C. Mouse chromosome 15 — Human chromosome 12
D. Mouse chromosome 2 — Human chromosome 2

All Hox genes have a number of features in common:

1. They all have homeoboxes at their three ends that are related to Drosophila homeotic gene homeoboxes.

2. They all have a single, small intron of 1 kb with homeobox being in the second exon.

3. They all have transcribed in the same direction.

They are all expressed in embryonic nervous system, somites and limbs.

34 Chapter

PAX GENES

Pax genes play key roles in the formation of tissues and organs during embryogenesis. Pax 3 and Pax 7 mark myogenic progenitor cells and regulate their behavior and their entry into the program of skeletal muscle differentiation. Recent results have underlined the importance of the Pax 3 and 7 population of cells for skeletal muscle development and regeneration.

The paired box genes are a family of nine developmental control genes, which in humans (PAX) and mice (Pax) encode nuclear transcription factors. The temporal and spatial expressions of these highly conserved genes are tightly regulated during foetal development including organogenesis.

PAX/Pax genes are switched off during the terminal differentiation of most structures. Specific mutations within a number of PAX/Pax genes lead to developmental abnormalities in both humans and mouse.

Mutation in PAX 3 causes Waardenburg syndrome, and craniofacial-deafness-hand syndrome. The Splotch phenotype in mouse exhibits defects in neural crest derivatives such as, pigment cells, sympathetic ganglia and cardiac neural crest-derived structures. The PAX family also plays key roles in several human malignancies. In particular, PAX 3 is involved in rhabdomyosarcoma and tumors of neural crest origin, including melanoma and neuroblastoma. This review critically evaluates the roles of PAX/Pax in oncogenesis. It especially highlights recent advances in knowledge of how their genetic alterations directly interfere in the transcriptional networks that regulate cell differentiation, proliferation, migration and survival and may contribute to oncogenesis.

Within the mammalian family, there are four well defined groups of Pax genes:

a. Pax group 1 (Pax 1 & 9)

b. Pax group 2 (Pax 2, 5 & 8)

c. Pax group 3 (Pax 3 & 7)

d. Pax group 4 (Pax 4 & 6)

Pax gene that contains a DNA binding domain similar to one in the paired genes of Drosophila. Eight Pax genes have been identified in Drosophila and nine Pax genes in mammals, which have been identified and most of them are expressed in the nervous system during development.

Pax genes encode a complex family of transcription factors with multiple DNA-binding domains and diverse functions and for this reason many of the aspects of their evolution remain speculative. Pax genes are defined by the presence of paired box which was first identified in the Drosophila.

In human beings, the paired box containing (PAX) gene family, only two members – PAX – 3 and PAX – 6, have been found to be associated with Waardenburg's syndrome and aniridia respectively and they have been mapped to human chromosomes.

35

Chapter

Sox Genes

Sox genes are defined as containing the HMG box of a gene involved in sex determination called SRY which resides on the Y- chromosome. (Sox = SRY related HMG box).

Approximately about 30 SOX genes have been identified. Almost all SOX genes show at least 50 percent amino acid similarity with the HMG box in SRY.

The Sox family of genes are important in the development of an individual but they do not have single function. Many members have the ability to regulate several different aspects of development.

They are important in the process of neuronal development and determination of sex. It is thought that some Sox genes may be useful in the early diagnosis of childhood brain tumors. For example Sox 2 and Sox 3 are involved in the transition between epithelial granule cells in the cerebellum to their migratory state. Granule cells differentiate to granule neurons, with Sox 11 being involved in this process.

Sox 4 is a transcription factor in lymphocytes (B and T) and is required for B lymphocyte development.

The SOX genes thus control organ development. Mutations of these genes cause human genetic diseases including dwarfism, testicular cancer and possibly diabetes and other severe clinical consequences.

Much like an electrical circuit, SOX genes/SOX factors exist as networks, switching on or off, leading to the formation of different organs and tissues during the development of the embryo.

36

Chapter

DNA HYBRIDIZATION

DNA HYBRIDIZATION

The pairing of two DNA molecules, often form two different sources by hydrogen bonding between complementary nucleotides. The technique frequently used to detect presence of a specific nucleotide sequence in a DNA sample.

DNA PROBE

Segment of DNA that is labeled (tagged) so that after a DNA hybridization reaction, any basic pairing between probe and a complementary base sequence in a DNA sample can be detected.

DNA is made up of many nucleotides. The target nucleotide sequence in a DNA sample can be determined with a probe. This procedure is called DNA hybridization. The procedure depends on formation of a stable base pair between DNA probe and targeted nucleotide sequence.

DNA hybridization is feasible because double stranded DNA can be converted into single stranded DNA by heat or alkali treatment. Heating DNA breaks hydrogen bonds that hold bases together. (DENATURATION), but does affect phosphodiester bond of DNA backbone. If the heated solution is rapidly cooled, the strand remain single. But if heated solution is slowly cooled, double stranded helical conformation of DNA can be restricted because of base pairing of complementary nucleotides (RENATURATION). This process of heating and slowly cooling double stranded DNA is called ANNEALING. When DNA from different sources with some shared sequences are mixed, heated to 100°C and slowly cooled, there will be some hybrid DNA molecules among the annealed products, i.e., double stranded DNA molecules in which strand come from different sources.

The target DNA is denatured and single stranded DNA are irreversibly bond to a matrix, i.e., Nitrocellulose or Nylon. This binding is carried out at high speed temperature. Then single strands of DNA probe which are labeled with either a radioisotope or another tag system, and are incubated with bound DNA sample. If the sequence of nucleotide in the DNA probe is complementary to a nucleotide sequence in the sample, then base pairing that is hybridization occurs. The hybridization can be detected by autoradiography or visualization procedures depending upon nature of DNA probe label. If the nucleotide sequence of probe does not base pair with a DNA sequence in the sample, then hybridization occurs.

Generally probe range in length from 100 to more than 1000 bp, although both larger and smaller probes can be used. Stable base pairing require a match of >80% with a segment of 50 bases.

Scheme

1. Bind single stranded DNA (target) to a membrane support.
2. Add single stranded labeled DNA (probe) under appropriate conditions of temperature and ionic strength to promote base pairing between the two.
3. Wash the support to remove excess unbound labeled probe DNA.
4. Detect the hybrid sequence that forms between probe and target DNA.

It has three elements: Probe DNA, target DNA and signal detection.

The detection system is sensitive and specific, e.g., faecal matter, urine, blood samples, throat wash, tissue samples without extensive DNA purification are used.

In most research labs nucleic acid hybridization is routinely detected by labeling the probe with a radioactive isotope–Phosphorous-32.

Radiolabel led probe is mixed with target DNA that is bound to the membrane support. After it is washed free of non-hybridized probe DNA, presence of radioactivity is determined by lying the membrane on X-ray film (autoradiography). Phosphorous-32 is potentially dangerous, short lived, needs safe handling and disposing.

Non radioactive system for indicating hybrid DNA formation has also been developed. Normally biotin-labeled nucleotides incorporated into DNA probe. Advantages of it are: it is stable at least for a year at room temperature and as sensitive as radioactive one.

GENETIC CLONING

The term cloning refers, in general to making multiple copies of something.

Identical twins are whole body clones of each other.

Genetic cloning is multiple copies of molecules at DNA level (molecular clones).

For the purpose researchers need extraordinary tiny samples of DNA which may be impure, fragmented or ancient.

The scientists are now learning how to deal with DNA extracted from pathology collections, old and dusty museum exhibits, archaeological specimens such as Egyptian mummies and extinct animals. They may start with DNA present in the cells at the base of a single human hair.

The process of cloning begins with the polymerase chain reaction (PCR).

Essentially PCR singles out a stretch of about 50 to 2000 nucleotides from the total DNA present in a sample and multiplies this target DNA million fold or more in just 4 hours.

Thus starting with one or a few copies of target DNA, investigators can rapidly amplify it enough to do whatever analysis are called for.

To use it, researchers must already know the order of at least 20 nucleotides at each end of the target region.

A complimentary base pairing is used as a kind of glue. It was thus possible to insert DNA from primitive frog, Xenopus into DNA of E. coli, where the frog DNA subsequently reproduced itself as if it were at home.

Plasmids are used as vehicles to carry the DNA molecules inserted into the cell.

Instead of plasmids other vectors can be introduced into E. coli, example, bacteriophage. Cosmids, because they accommodate more pieces of foreign DNA than plasmids.

Organisms other than E. coli are also used for cloning and that is, Baker's yeast. This organism is easily grown and manipulated in laboratory glassware and can be maintained in haploid or diploid state. Moreover, yeast is a eukaryotic organism. Fertilized egg of mammal is also used for cloning.

DNA thus introduced, keeps multiplying in the vector and forms various useful proteins.

When vector DNA is enlarged by the addition of a piece of foreign DNA it becomes a vehicle for transporting foreign DNA into other E. coli cells. The recipient bacteria are treated with calcium chloride which alters the cell wall and permits an occasional plasmid or vector to enter. The foreign DNA now starts replicating and has been cloned just as in polymerase chain reaction.

Advantages

1. Manipulation of DNA helps in correcting the abnormal sequences of amino acid chains in DNA molecule. This is best used in repairing of dead tissue and gene therapy in various genetic disorders.
2. The extinct animals can be cloned to increase the population of those affected animals.
3. Insulin dependant diabetes mellitus can be cured by replacing missing gene concerned with insulin secretion.
4. Children with pituitary dwarfism, leukemia, AIDS related Kaposi sarcoma, warts, hepatitis C can be treated by replacing the missing factor or protein.
5. Cows and goats treated by human DNA encoding tPA produced milk rich in human enzyme tissue plasminogen activator (tPA) which is useful in prevention of heart attacks due to clot formation (dissolves clot).
6. Cloning of calf gives medicinal milk and milk protein.
7. Immortality of DNA is used to solve the crimes.
8. After cloning the animals the animal organs can be used as donors for tomorrow.

Disadvantages

Because bacteria are living cells, they not only replicate the genetic material but also transcribe it into messenger and translate it into polypeptide products.

The bacteria can do the same with foreign genes and alter them that may give rise to anomalous gene or anomalous individual.

Wrong decisions may be made during the process of cloning which may lead to ecological disaster or disaster in population, such as cloning in E. coli any DNA derived from known pathogens or cancer causing viruses.

Therefore, the genetic cloning should be used to manipulate for the betterment of mankind.

POLYMERASE CHAIN REACTION

It is a procedure in molecular biology wherein millions of copies of DNA from few copies or a single copy of that particular (specific region) DNA sequence is generated. It is the most important technique used in biotechnological and medical laboratories. Its uses are in DNA cloning, functional analysis of genes, identification of DNA based phylogeny, diagnosis of the hereditary diseases, identification of fingerprints in paternity testing, detection of infectious diseases and in gene therapy in various genetic disorders and various genetic manipulations. This technique was first performed in 1983 by Kary Mullis. The method consists of – DNA melting and enzymatic replication of short fragments of DNA called DNA primers. This procedure requires repeated heating and cooling of DNA fragments called 'thermal cycling'. The key components for repeated amplification are the short DNA fragments (primers) containing the sequences complementary to target region along with DNA polymerase. The new DNA copy thus generated is taken as a template for replication. This sets a chain reaction in which enormous copies of DNA are formed.

The heat stable DNA polymerase is used in all PCR applications. Some of the polymerases like 'Taq polymerase' is obtained from thermus aquaticus bacterium. The DNA polymerase assembles a new DNA strand from DNA oligonucleotides which form nucleotides required for DNA synthesis. The rate of amplification varies from 10 kilo base pairs (bp) to 40 kilo base pairs (bp).

Requirement of Basic PCR

1. DNA template which is to be amplified.
2. Two primers (short fragments of DNA called primers).
3. Taq polymerase with a temperature at around 70°C.
4. Building blocks from which DNA polymerase synthesizes new DNA strand.
5. Buffer solution for the provision of suitable chemical environment for optimum activity and stability of DNA polymerase.
6. Divalent cations like magnesium / manganese ions.
7. Monovalent cations like potassium ions.
   Volume of reaction tubes is 0.2 ml to 0.5 ml.

   The reaction volume 10–200 µl in a thermal cycle.

For about 20 to 30 seconds, changes or cycles are given with the temperature of 94 to 98°C. It is followed by cycles at about 50 to 65°C for 20 to 40 sec. These steps are repeated. This is done for about 1 to 9 minutes for heating (DNA melting) and cooling. This causes disruption of hydrogen bonds between the complimentary bases and yield single strands of DNA molecules. It also helps the hydrogen in DNA molecule to become stable. Then the primers are used to match the templates of DNA sequence. The polymerase binds to primer the template in that sequence which begins to synthesize DNA. The polymerase keeps on producing DNA which keeps on amplifying continuously. The synthesis of DNA is limited if there is use of limiting reagents or chemicals. At optimum temperature the DNA polymerase will polymerize thousand bases per minute.

The last step of elongation consists of last PCR cycles at the temperature of 70–74°C for 5 to15 minutes. Indefinite time may be employed at 4–15°C for short term storage.

COMET ASSAY (SCGE)

Comet assay is a technique which is highly sensitive and a simple technique in which the damage level of the DNA or the RNA at eukaryotic cell can be detected. The damages leading to mutations and decreased DNA repairs could be due to oxidation or methylation by the biological processes in cancers of colon, prostate, breast, neurological diseases like Alzheimer's disease, Parkinson's disease and dementia associated with Lewy bodies (abnormal aggregations of proteins in the cells) etc. Such damages could lead to susceptibility to cancer.

This technique is also called Single Cell Gel Electrophoresis (SCGE). This technique was first explained by Singh *et al.* in 1988. Now it has become one of the methods to evaluate the DNA damage or repair and genotoxicity testing. The basic principle behind this technique is that the cells are encapsulated in low melting point agarose gel suspension at 37° C, cause lysis of cells in neutral or alkaline conditions. The lysed cells are subjected to staining and electrophoresis of the cells (cell along with its nucleus). Visual analysis will be made for calculating fluorescence to assess the extent of the damage to the DNA or the RNA. This procedure can be performed both manually and by using imaging software for automatic and quick results.

Therefore this procedure involves four stages–they are: 1. Encapsulation, 2. Lysis, 3. Electrophoresis, and 4. Imaging or analysis.

In encapsulation, the cells obtained by cell culture or from the body are dispersed and suspended in the molten agarose gel, which has a low melting point, at 37°C. This suspension is cast on a glass slide used to fix it on microscope. Then a cover slip is put close to the suspension and the slide and cover slip are brought in contact. The slide is then tilted and the suspension is made to slide on the glass slide with the help of the cover slip till a thin film is obtained. As the thin layer is formed the agarose is allowed to be gelled at 4°C and the cover slip is removed. The agarose forms a matrix of osmotically neutral carbohydrate fibers. This encapsulation prevents the cells from shifting or distorting and simultaneously allows the solutions to penetrate into the cells. Now the cells are subjected to a test agent which causes the DNA damage in the encapsulated cells. Standardized level of DNA damage can be done by using hydrogen peroxide for calibration.

In lysis stage the slides are immersed into a highly concentrated salt solution or a detergent (Sarcosinate or Triton X–100). It is done at 4°C for one to two hours. The pH of the solution is either neutral or alkaline, depending upon the type of damage. The detergent dissolves the cell membrane and the aqueous salt solution causes damage to the cell membrane which is made up of protein. All the cellular contents except the DNA are destroyed and flow into the agarose matrix. DNA of the cell remains in the capsule of agarose and unravels to fill in the cavity of the agarose matrix where the entire cell was formerly occupying. This mass of DNA into the capsule of agarose is called 'nucleoid'. After 2 hours the slide is washed to remove the salt.

This stage is followed by Electrophoresis, wherein the slide is dipped into the electrophoresis solution with an adjusted pH, for about 20 minutes. In alkaline fluid the DNA becomes denatured and single stranded. Electric field is applied 1V per cm for about 20 minutes. The slides are neutralized to pH 7, stained with fluorescent stains which are DNA specific (ethidium bromide and propidium iodide) and analyzed with a fluorescent microscope with a digital camera attached to it.

In the last stage the fluorescent microscope containing the mounted slide is connected to a computer with image analysis software.

The results are analyzed depending upon the appearance of the DNA. The undamaged DNA retains a highly organized association with the matrix proteins in the nucleus. The damaged DNA shows disrupted organization and loses its compacted nature and thus relaxes which makes it to expand out of the cavity of agarose capsule. The undamaged DNA remains in the cavity of agarose capsule and damaged fragments move farther in that given period of time. Thus the amount of DNA which moves out of the cavity of the capsule is the measure of the amount of DNA damage in the cell. This DNA spread resembles a comet and therefore it is also called comet assay. The brighter and longer the tail of the comet the higher is the damage level.

The damage to the DNA can be caused by ultraviolet rays, oxidation, cancer etc.

EUGENICS

This word is derived from Greek that means "well born".

According to Webster's New Universal Unabridged Dictionary: It is defined as 'the science that deals with the improvement of human race, breeds in case of animals through the control of hereditary factors. It is to get improving human genetic qualities by improving gene pool'.

It was by the human about two million years ago for the dog as a domestic animal, used for hunting, a loyal companion, for warning against the unknown people or objects. For these purpose a larger dog was needed. Therefore they had to choose a larger breed of dogs were selected for the larger dogs.

Every human is visualized as equal at birth, in beauty, mental and physical health, intelligence and social strength; that requires an evolutionary system with aims and plenty of planning for a healthy society.

Apart from the good quality breeds of animals like dogs, horses, pigs etc it is also concerned with prevention or elimination of genetic disorders like hemophilia, Huntington's disease, sickle cell anemia, malaria, tuberculosis etc. which are also influenced by the environment. Some of the genetic disabilities are compatible with life but some of them are lethal. Therefore some policies are needed for the improvement in the population. The policies are of two types – one is positive and the other is negative eugenic policy. The positive polices encourage reproduction among genetically normal individuals. The factors involved in bringing out such policies require financial support, political stimuli, in vitro fertilization, ovum transplants, cloning and analysis of the observations. The negative eugenics is targeted at lowering the reproduction among the genetically unsound couple. This is achieved by discouraging the sexual life for the genetically disadvantaged ones, medical terminations of pregnancy in case of conception, sterilization and various methods of family planning. But in many countries and many religions the prenatal diagnosis and medical termination of pregnancy or abortions are considered illegal. During 20th century many countries introduced genetic screening, marriage restrictions, segregation of mentally ill from the rest of the population, compulsory sterilization and genetic counseling.

The implementation methods are of three types:

1. **Mandatory eugenics (Authoritarian eugenics):** Where mandatory programs are planned for execution. For this, policies and legislation are involved in enforcing the mandate.

2. **Promotional eugenics:** It is voluntarily practiced and promoted to general population and it is not mandated officially. This requires a democratic or liberal approach.
3. **Voluntary eugenics:** It is neither a governmental program nor a private organization which is enforcing the population but it is purely voluntary and practiced by individuals or groups.

Eugenicists are of the opinion that the persons with low intelligent quotient are prevented from immigration to other countries. This leads to unethical issues and practices. Therefore corrective procedures are to be implemented for the benefit of the disadvantageous groups in the population.

Gradually animal husbandry was established for the consistent source of food, well-nourished animals/cattle for better quality milk and meat, stronger animals for transportation and later for entertainment like horse races, camel races etc., this was extended to the better quality growth of vegetables and fruits for the people in the society. Then came the cloning. The first clone was with a sheep. Human cloning is also possible but with lot of procedure, expenditure and complications. In case of female, the mitochondrial DNA (mtDNA) will influence the growing embryo.

INVESTING IN THE FUTURE

If the human society survives its current degeneration due to natural evolution long enough, eugenics will be developed and applied, even though no concerted species wide effort is made. It may take an extended time, perhaps 500 to 1,000 years, a significant period in light of the rate of human degeneration. If the society collapses before the underlying causes are recognized and corrected, then the species will become extinct.

Electronics (computers and such) is the current economic growth field. Medicine is also growing at a fast clip. The new field, however, one that will in time eclipse all of these, is molecular genetics. Modified, special purpose, life forms are being developed. Current experimentation includes hybrid biological/electronic devices, biological computer memories and research leading to the minimum molecular complexity for life. Creation of new life forms directly from biological raw (non-living) materials are quite possible in the near future.

The genome project has been enlightening. The human genome is being mapped. Current work on this project carries little resemblance to that envisioned when it started. Hundreds, perhaps thousands, of new techniques, ways of looking at the problem, solutions to problems not even realized before starting, have poured from the inventive minds working on it. But knowing its construction is a long way from knowing the functions within it, and how to correct it or improve on it.

A human culture is capable, when faced with a cause of sufficient importance, of a culture wide concerted effort. Witness the US during WWII and the subsequent cold war. An effort equal in scope to our military since WWII over a similar time period would provide the technical infrastructure for negating natural evolution and correcting the human genetic structure throughout the world, a gift from the US to every living human.

It would be a great adventure, collecting the finest human minds and providing them with the facilities to eliminate a sizable portion of all the ills the human is now afflicted with. We are capable of doing it to kill people, why not do it for the sake of saving an endangered species.

Index

Index